THe NarcissisT Slayer

by

Bev Baker

Published by New Generation Publishing in 2023

Front cover design by Max Andon
Proofreading and Editing: James Leder

First Edition

ISBN: 978-1-80369-776-5

www.newgeneration-publishing.com

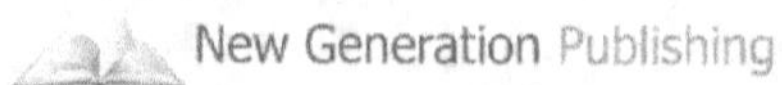

The characters in this book are fictitious and bear no resemblance to anyone alive or dead, yet the characters in this book are real and bear every resemblance to anyone who has ever had their life ripped apart by a narcissist.

THE ZOOM CALL

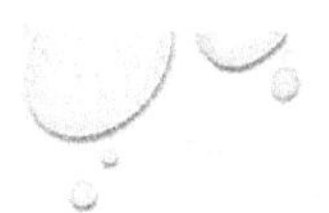

- WELCOME
- INTRODUCTIONS
- ITINERARY
- PROGRAMME
- TREATMENTS
- SELF CARE

"Hey everyone. Welcome. For those who don't know me, I am Bev and I am your host for next week's workshop. I am so glad you could join me today. Please put your videos on so that we can put names to faces and get to know each other a little more. I hope everyone can see the PowerPoint. Let's go through next week's agenda so you can see what the workshop is all about. If you have any questions whatsoever please don't hesitate to ask.

You have signed up to the Narcissist Workshop. Congratulations. You have signed up most likely because you are sick to death with dealing with a narcissist.

You've probably done all the right things, but still the narcissist lives in your head. Rent free! They define your every move. You want it to stop. You want to heal and get on with your life. Am I right?"

They all nodded.

"Good! On Sunday we will all be in the beautiful island of Malta. Malta has everything: sun, sea, sand, good food and lovely people.

You will just have to take my word for it there will be no time for sightseeing. If you want to see Malta then put it on your bucket list. We are on the island of Malta to slay dragons and not to frolic.

A word of warning. If you have signed up to this workshop to gather tips and tricks on how to get back at the narcissist, you're on the wrong workshop. I am happy to give you your money back. If you think you have joined this workshop so you can outwit your narcissist, then think again. I am happy to give you your money back. One more thing: if you think this is a cosy workshop by the sea, where you can engage in a 'pity party' and sing 'Kumbaya' at night, then think again. I am more than happy to give you your money back. I want you to be under no illusion what the workshop is about. We are going to slay dragons and you need to be ready.

Introductions

You all know me and you will find out how I work on the workshop. I would love to hear from you at this point. Please unmute yourselves, introduce yourselves to the rest of the group and tell us what you want to get out of the workshop. I would be grateful if you could be brief. I don't want us to go into specifics here because we will cover everything next week in detail.

Who would like to go first?"

There was an awkward silence.

"I'll go first. Get it out the way. My name is Cynthia. I have watched nearly all of your videos on TikTok and you have helped me realise that I am not the crazy one. I am so excited, I can't tell you. I am dealing with a narcissist who has ruined my life. I know I need to move on but I can't get him out of my head. How did this happen to me? I am banking on this workshop giving me answers".

"Thank you, Cynthia, and welcome. You will get answers, I guarantee it".

"Hi everyone. My name is Harshida. I have been living with a narcissist sociopath arsehole for 22 years now. I have been leaving him every year for the past 22 years. I have washed, cooked, cleaned and iron his fucking shirts for too long. I am little more than a glorified slave. Let me take that back. I am not a glorified slave. I am a fucking slave. I need to gather what little I have of myself left and do something about my life. I am here because I have had enough and I am desperate. Oh and I swear a lot. Forgive me"

"Welcome Harshida. Thank you".

"So I am James, forty seven years of age. Hi everyone. My ex is the narcissist. My son lives with her. It tears me up inside to know what's going on. My son tells me about her, but I feel as if I can't say anything because if I do she will take it out on him. She calls me and screams

down the phone and then she blocks me before I can say anything. She is making my life a living hell. I don't know what is best to do. I cannot understand how a mother can use her own child as a weapon against me. I do not want my son to suffer because of me. I need to make sense of what is happening. I hope this workshop will give me answers".

"Thank you James for sharing. Your position is a tough one. Many people are in a similar predicament as you. It is complicated and during the workshop I will give you as many tools as I can muster to empower you to deal with it. I promise you. Who's next?"

"Me. Hello everyone. I am Fosia. I am the victim of narcissistic abuse. The narcissist has cleaned out my bank account. He went through my savings like a locust. The worst thing of all is that I let him. How could I let this happen to me? I am so ashamed of myself. But do you know what the worst thing about this is? I can't stop thinking about him. I drive myself crazy wondering where he is, what he's doing and who he's doing it with. That's mad. After all he's put me through, I can't get him out of my head. I look in the mirror and I don't recognise myself. What I want from this workshop is to find myself again".

They could feel Fosia's pain. Even on Zoom. Her distress spoke for them all.

"Thank you Fosia. Don't worry, you'll get through this. Who's next?"

"Good afternoon. My name is William. I came across a random podcast which explained the narcissist. I felt as if someone had just read my life story to me. It was an 'aha' moment and an 'oh no' moment all at once. I want the workshop to help me make sense of what happened to me, show me who I am and give me some tools so that I can move on with my life".

"No pressure then William. I'll certainly do my best. Next?"

"Hi, Sarah here. I don't even know where to start. My mother is a narcissist. Your videos have showed me that it isn't my imagination and I am not the one who is crazy. I have so many questions.

Since I was spawned by the devil, am I a narcissist? Does narcissism run in families? I feel that my mother ruined my life. I make bad choices. I try to please everyone. I go out of my way to please others and they never think about me. In fact most people shit on me from a great height. I am usually the afterthought for everyone. Why do I attract narcissists? I am on this workshop because I want to know what I'm doing wrong".

"Thank you Sarah."

"I'll go next. Hi people. I am VJ and I was raised by wolves. I am jesting, but it feels like that. My family are aliens to me and I am an alien to them. My parents have tried to define who I am and

who I should be all my life. I have well and truly had enough. I need to be 'me' but I have no clue who 'me' is. I need to find out who I am or at least get some pointers that will help me to discover who I am".

"I'm last. Hi everyone my name is Geordie. My mother is a narcissist. I have gone 'no contact' but I can't get away from her. As you said earlier, Bev, she lives rent free in my head. It's like having a lodger in your house but you pay their rent. I am done trying to sweep shit under the carpet or pretending that things that matter don't matter. It's exhausting! I am ready to make sense of the abuse I suffered as a child, if that is possible. I am on this workshop because I need all the help I can get to become the person I was supposed to be before my mother got a hold of me. I have high hopes for this workshop".

"So do I Geordie, so do I. Well, thank you all for introducing yourselves. I know that couldn't have been easy. By the way swearing and using curse words is not a prerequisite for the workshop but it helps".

They laughed a little too long and a little too hard. Nerves.

"Contrary to popular belief, swearing can be liberating. Sometimes, when you are describing what happened to you or what you are going through, only a swear word will do. Society tells us that it isn't good form to swear. It is the same society that tells us not to talk about abuse. It is interesting to me that people get offended by swear words and they are not offended by the narcissist who systematically fucks up people's lives. In the workshop, you will have the opportunity to tell your story and if it takes a stream of swear words to do so, so be it.

All of you are strangers now, but let me tell you something: by the end of the workshop, you will have bonded like nothing you have experienced before. True bonding. You will bond with your stories, through your pain and in your dogged determination to heal and find happiness. I am here for that.

Let's go over the itinerary. If you have any questions then please ask. If you think of a question after this call then please email Bevtalks@outlook.com.

Itinerary

As I said, we are holding the workshop on the beautiful island of Malta. Asia will be at the airport to pick you up and take you to the resort. She will be standing in arrivals with a huge yellow umbrella. You cannot miss her. The sole reason for the Sunday arrival is so that you can settle in smoothly. All the tourists seem to arrive on a Monday morning and we would waste a lot of time if we get caught up with them. So when you arrive at the resort on Sunday soak up the atmosphere. Familiarise yourselves with the layout. You have a map of the resort in your pack and you will see that the all the key areas are well signposted. You will not get lost. Dinner is served between 6.30 and 9pm every evening.

The programme

The workshop starts at 10 am and will finish around 4 pm.

Monday, Tuesday all day and Thursday morning the workshop will be at the Beach House in the resort.

On Wednesday, the workshop will be held on the beach. The resort has a beautiful cove area on the beach about 30 minutes' walk. We will meet at reception at 9am on Wednesday morning and walk to the cove together. Don't worry about anything, the resort has taken care of everything. There will be food and drink obviously, sun loungers and chairs and parasols. All you need to do is wear sensible shoes, bring sun cream and a hat. I'll tell you more about it when the time comes. On Thursday we will have the morning session, lunch and then Asia will take you back to the airport. Please check out in the morning so that you don't get charged for an extra day. Leave your luggage at reception or bring it with you to the workshop. Make sure you are ready to leave at 2pm.

The programme is not rigid. You are the programme. I had to start somewhere, right? I am your host and I am going to be a good host. Firm but fair. I do not want you to go away from this call thinking that you are going to go through a baptism of fire next week. On the contrary, this course has been designed to be joyous. The only one that gets burnt is the narcissist. As far as you are concerned, you are the phoenix from the ashes. You'll see.

Treatments

In the workshop you will learn a lot more about the narcissist which is empowering in itself because you will develop a new awareness and have many 'aha' moments. At the same time, it is important to release trauma from your body. How you do this is through body work. I recommend that if you are not actually in the workshop with the rest of us then you should be either having a treatment, taking an exercise class or doing some sort of activity. Trauma attaches itself to every cell of your body and can make you sick. Every cell in your body needs to heal. Healing is not a theoretical exercise. I don't know who said that time is a healer. They are wrong. There are people who are still suffering from trauma and PTSD twenty years after their encounter with their abuser. Some people never recover. Healing doesn't occur by osmosis. Healing is a process and it is flipping hard work.

Try as many things as you can. Take a dance class, give acupuncture or cranial head therapy a go. Learn to meditate while you are here. It will help you sleep. Have as many different types of massage as you can.

I need to talk about water. Water is your friend. Swimming is a great way to de-stress and reset the brain. When you swim the brain gets to do what it was designed to do which is keeping you alive.

If you can go out into the sea and swim or even splash around, all the better. The cold water is a great way to detox your system. If you can't stand the cold then go the other way. Take advantage of the Turkish baths and the sauna. What I'm saying is that any kind of spa activity will accelerate your healing. When you are not in the water then make sure you drink plenty of water.

SeLF-Care

I will say that the workshop is intense at times. I am not going to lie. It's going to be tough going for all of you at some point and at different points. The first thing you must do is take care of yourself. Let me tell you when we get going I will often forget to take a break. The only time I will say 'break' is if it is a good time to change topics not because I think you need caffeine. Breaks are twenty minutes long.

It is up to you to stay hydrated, to go to the bathroom or to get up and stretch your legs. Put yourselves first.

When you go on a flight the first thing the air steward says is to fasten your own safety belt. You are of no use to anyone if you are bumping around all over the place. In fact you may be a danger. The idea of putting yourself first may seem selfish. Good! It may feel awkward at first. Work with it, you'll get used to it! Looking after yourself is how you build healthy boundaries and you need to build boundaries so that no narcissist, past, present or future can creep into your life and take liberties.

Although I have spoken to each of you and I am aware of your medical history, I am not a doctor and so the onus is on you to take care of yourself. If you are on any medication whatsoever then please continue to take it. You will feel different in this workshop and you may feel inspired to throw out your medication. Don't do that. If after the workshop you want to come off your meds then wait until you get back and discuss it with your doctor.

I want all of you to feel safe in the knowledge that whatever we talk about remains between all of us. You are on this workshop and not the narcissist. The workshop is all about you and your recovery. You will take the narcissist with you to Malta, you will deal with them in Malta and you will leave them there. You will return to your country, narcissist free. It goes without saying that the workshop is strictly confidential. Every word that is spoken amongst us in Malta stays in Malta. I hope I have your agreement on this.

Oh one last thing. There is 'wifi' at the resort but you will not be needing it.

If you have any further questions about anything at all then do not hesitate to contact us at bevtalks@outlook.com. I think you will find that

Asia has taken care of everything so that you have a wonderful experience. Asia is your customer service contact and event planner for this workshop. If you have a problem she will fix it.

So that's it, I will see you in Malta. Safe flight everyone!

This call has ended.

MONDAY

Bev had been cleansing in the Beach House for at least 30 minutes. It was something she did for every workshop. Rooms had memories. If rooms and buildings could talk they would have a lot of jaw-dropping things to say.

Bev worked with energy. She could pick up vibrations. It was often problematic when she stayed in hotels. All sorts of things happened in hotels. People have arguments and say horrible things in hotel rooms. People use hotel rooms to hide from people. People use hotel rooms to carry out their secret affairs. People commit suicide in hotel rooms. Her beloved teacher, an amazing clinical psychologist, had booked a hotel room, drunk a bottle of brandy, taken a fistful of pills and ended her own life. The memory of her teacher holding court at one of her lectures flashed before her eyes. What this woman didn't know about mental health issues was nobody's business. Yet with all her knowledge she couldn't save herself.

A couple of times when she had been too tired or it was too late to change rooms she had stayed in a room and suffered sleep paralysis. It was as if someone or something was holding her down. It was petrifying. She mentioned it to a friend who was a priest and he had told her that if it happened again she should make the sign of the cross with her tongue. She did it and it worked.

She brought herself back to the task at hand. Whenever she went into an environment to stay she made sure that she purified the space. She purified the room with sage the herb, moved the chairs around to shake up the energy and opened up all the windows so that the crisp sea air could fill the room. The music she had selected also did its job. She always chose uplifting music.

'Thunder' from the band Imagine Dragons filled the air.

"I was lightening before the thunder...

Thunder   thunder...lightening   before   the thunder...thun...thun

Thunder thunder...lightening before the thunder"

She loved the song. It was her theme tune and her war cry.

Image the creativity that any artist puts into their work. She wanted that vibration to be present today. The space looked beautiful. It had lovely cosy chairs, drinks and snacks on tap and the most wonderful views. The beach created an amazing backdrop. Bev paused to take in the scenery. Far in the distance she could make out fishermen preparing their boats to go out to sea. She finished off the look of the space with a lovely bunch of yellow flowers she had picked up in the local market the day before.

Bev is a claircognizant. It is one of the four major intuitive gifts. Most people are aware of clairvoyance, clairaudience and clairsentience, but not a lot of people are aware of claircognizance.

Claircognizance literally translated means 'clear knowing'. In other words, you just know stuff without knowing how you know or why you know. You could call it intuition or gut instinct. Everyone has intuition to a greater or lesser degree but most people don't use it. Even when the signs are obvious, people still don't follow their instincts. Why? Fear.

Being a claircognizant was a gift.

She could heal people quickly. She didn't have to ask, she knew as soon as she saw them. When her clients realised that she got it they invariably cried with relief. The first step to healing is being heard and to be taken seriously. She only needed to hear a person's story once and she knew everything. She could feel pain.

She loved what Einstein said:

"Everything is energy and that's all there is to it". Energy cannot be destroyed, it can only be transmuted. And that was it in a nutshell. Her job was moving energies around.

People loved to tell their stories again and again. This she called 'stuckness'. This happened when the person was stuck in the past and too afraid to move on. The more they repeated the same story the more gripping the story becomes. Every time someone told their story the more twists and turns it revealed. They wouldn't let go. The story defined them. It shaped their every move. She had learned a few fancy moves to get people to detach from their stories: hypnotherapy, guided meditations, tarot cards and NLP. What had got Bev into mental health was Transactional Analysis. Transactional Analysis is the study of personality and communication. Eric Berne, the developer of Transactional Analysis, had often said that you could tell everything about a person within the first five minutes of meeting them. Simply by the things they said and the way that they say the things they say. She had spent the best part of four years simply analysing words and meaning. She was expert at analysing transactions. She only allowed her clients to tell their story once. After that it was healing time. Her only job was to encourage her clients to show up to their own lives.

For her the words that people use were the end of the trail. The words give way to thoughts and patterns of thinking. The patterns of thinking give way to beliefs and values. The values give way to identity. It was her experience that when someone has been through a traumatic event, it is their identity – their sense of who they are- that needs to be healed. What a person deep down thinks and feels about themselves colours the way that they present themselves to the world.

Just like every empath, she could feel pain. Going into London was a tough gig for her. There were so many homeless people on the streets. It was unbearable. She always carried loose change to give. Many of her friends mocked her and argued that the homeless would only use the money to buy drugs. They missed the point. Bev could feel the person's discomfort as they adjusted their butt cheeks against the stone cold pavement. She could feel their loss of dignity. She could feel the emotional spark of rejection when the homeless person made eye contact with another human and that human looked away. But everything is energy and the people who turn away from suffering do not get away with it either, they think they do but they don't. There was a shock of guilt and shame for turning away. There was a bolt of anger for being confronted with so much suffering on a daily basis. She felt the inevitable build up of cognitive dissonance midst the stories they told themselves about the homeless in order to feel better about themselves.

She knew why many of the homeless had dogs. They are barcly able to feed themselves and yet many of them have a dog that needs feeding. It is a fact of life that everyone from the streets to the palace needs to feel as if they matter to someone.

Bev had a dog. Apart from getting supplies, her dog was the major reason why she left the house.

She had long ago given up going anywhere where there were a lot of people. She could hear the conversations people had with themselves inside their heads. It was usually negative.

Shops were her worst nightmare. She could pick up people's quiet desperation.

"I shouldn't buy this, I can't afford it".

"Damn it's too small. I'll buy it and it will give me an incentive to slim into it".

"It doesn't suit me. I'm so ugly...out of shape...so fucking fat."

"It doesn't look the same on me as it does on the model."

Thoughts are waves of brain energy. People don't realise that the way they think is written all over their faces and bodies.

Thoughts become words. Words are particles. Words direct behaviour. A repeated behaviour forms a habit and a habit becomes a way of life.

Being a claircognizant wasn't easy. She couldn't go to the movies. She didn't listen to the news. She didn't have to, she already knew. It was a human condition to spread bad news.

She realised over time and after lot of struggle that in order to be a decent claircognizant she had to stay clear of people. Otherwise her thoughts became contaminated. In order to be a decent claircognizant you need to be clear and being around people with their emotions seeping all over the place made her life very difficult. She lived off grid. Even in London it's possible.

These days she called herself a mental health coach. But that wasn't it. She had long ago stopped referring to herself as a 'therapist'. When people knew she was a therapist they either avoided her or wanted free therapy. She had learnt long ago that if people got stuff for free then they never valued it. She was reminded of a wonderful experiment where a famous virtuoso gave a free concert in a subway somewhere in the States. He barely made a hundred dollars in tips. Yet that night he gave the same concert to a packed out audience where each ticket cost more than a hundred dollars.

She was known as a trainer in certain circles and had worked for some big renowned companies. She was a writer, a coach and a motivational speaker. You name it. She had dipped her toe in almost everything to do with the development of people. She didn't want to call herself a healer. To her that was pompous. Yet that was what she was. She was a healer. In recent times she had become a social media influencer. This title was bemusing to her. The way that she had become a social media influencer was surreal.

On the day before Will Smith decided to end his career at the Oscars by slapping Chris Rock on live TV, she woke up knowing she had to post something about narcissism to her 369 followers on TikTok. The next day she was told that the video had gone viral. She didn't even know what going viral meant. But her videos kept going viral. Victims of narcissistic abuse came out of the woodwork. Virtually overnight she had hundreds of thousands of followers and millions of likes and views. It was mind blowing to her.

The group had met up briefly in the bar last night. Asia had attended to their every need. Soft pillow. Hard pillow. Vegetarian meals. She wasn't there to meet and greet them in the bar. She never was. She knew that they would be full of trepidation and she didn't want any of that nervous energy to take hold. She knew that if she showed up there would be a million questions.

"What time's lunch?"

"Do you think the narcissist I'm dealing with is a special case?"

"What would you do in this situation?"

She didn't want to start the workshop in the bar on a Sunday night.

The group came en masse. They had bonded. It was good to see.

They got coffee and eventually sat down. If fear had a colour it would be brown. They all looked as if they had pooped their pants.

"Good morning"!

There was no reply. There never was.

"Don't be afraid. You are in safe hands. I want to commend you all for attending this workshop. It means that you are fighters. It means that you are willing to do the work to be free. And that's what this workshop is all about.

Now I know that you have already shared your stories. What else are you going to do in a resort bar on a Sunday evening - drink and tell your stories? Right!

On this workshop we are going to mix it up. We are not going to dwell on the stories. After all, you know your own story. You have been telling yourself the same story over and over again. Telling your story over and over and dissecting it piece by piece doesn't solve the problem. In fact telling your story to yourself and to anyone who will listen reinforces the story. Every time you tell it you remember something different. Every time you tell the story you embellish it. Every time you tell the story you give power to the story and the abuser. The story is all-consuming. It defines you. You cannot move beyond your story. Every time you tell your story you are training your brain to be a victim. On this workshop you will get the opportunity to tell your story only once and then I hope you decide to put the story down and start to tell a different story.

With the end in mind we will approach the workshop back to front. Today and tomorrow we are going to talk about the narcissist. You need to know everything about them. Once you know everything there is to know about the narcissist you will only be a victim if you choose to be. Knowledge is power and only when you are equipped with the power of knowledge do you get to tell your story to all of us.

On Wednesday you will tell your story at the cove on the beach and you will leave your story there, on the beach. When you walk back to the resort you will feel light, free and on the path to healing. You will find that in the light of knowledge your story must change. It has to change. Those are the laws of science. When you observe something deeply, it changes.

Once you know differently you are empowered to do things differently. On Thursday we will have a couple of hours together to wrap up the workshop. You will be on your way to the airport by 2 o'clock. Leave your bags at reception or by all means bring them here.

So without further ado let's begin.

I was walking my dog not too long ago and I overheard a conversation. The person on the phone had been accused of gaslighting a mutual friend and they were talking about gaslighting as if they were ordering pepperoni on a pizza. I was so tempted to tell them that everything they think they know about gaslighting was wrong.

It struck me that everyone is an expert on narcissism these days. Any dodgy behaviour from anyone and the human cry is 'narcissist'. Johnny

Depp. Amber Hurd. Jada Pinkett-Smith. All of the Kardashians. Adam Levine. Every actor in Hollywood. The Cuomo brothers. Donald Trump. Boris Johnson. Liz Truss. Vladimir Putin. In fact anyone can be called out as a narcissist these days. We could blame social media for this. But is social media to blame or has social media simply brought shitty behaviour to our attention?

Just because someone posts selfies every five minutes does that make them a narcissist? Are we confusing vanity with narcissism? I don't believe you can turn a person into a narcissist unless they were a closet narcissist in the first place. Yes it is true, social media is the narcissist's playground, but at the same time social media has helped a lot of people just like you.

I bet you had no idea that narcissism was a thing but narcissism existed long before social media. We just didn't have a word to describe it. Abuse isn't new. People have suffered at the hands of others since humans have been on the planet. Domestic violence has always been there. Toxic and dysfunctional relations have always been there. Child abuse has always been there. Egotistical, arrogant, entitled, selfish shitty behaviour has always been here. We just have a word for it now and the word is narcissism.

The Making of the Narcissist

For some reason which evades me, we humans are fascinated with bad behaviour. I bet you if you go to Netflix right now you will see movie after movie about the narcissist, sociopath or psychopath. I have never seen a movie where the protagonist is a schizophrenic or suffers with OCD. Why doesn't Spielberg or Tarrantino direct a movie where the main character suffers with eating disorders? Maybe it's because eating disorders aren't sexy; the narcissist is the real deal reaction.

The narcissist is also big business. We are entertained by the antics of the narcissist. The narcissist scams, catfishes and takes people for a complete ride. We love it. We can't get enough of '90 day Fiancé', 'The Bachelor', 'Love Island', 'Married at First Sight' to name but a few and we love the drama. We can see what's going on and yet we are addicted. We think that what we see on these psychodrama programmes masquerading as reality TV could never happen to us. We are fooling ourselves when in actuality the same shit is happening to us in real time right under our nose. You think that if those beautiful people can put up with such shitty behaviour then 'who am I' to complain. We think that by watching such drama we can appease ourselves that others have it worse than us. Underneath it all, real reason we are fascinated by other people's drama instead of focusing on our own drama is hope. Yes, we hope that the eighty five year old with the one tooth in their head and the twenty five year old with the wandering eye find love. We hope that there is love at first sight and that they don't notice that the person they have travelled half way across the world to be with has no neck. You hope that they will pick out their one true love out of twenty gorgeous beings each carrying a rose. We hope that when they confess their deepest fears to the stranger they have just married in full view of a camera crew and a global audience that everything will work out rarely fine in the end. Even though it never ever does work out we still hope. We think that the narcissist will never happen to us until the narcissist happens to us.

CLUSteր B

All mental health issues that we know about are categorised and listed in the DSM-5. The DSM-5 or Diagnostic Statistical Manual, 5th edition is the tool used by mental health professionals to diagnose mental illnesses and conditions. Narcissism is listed as a personality disorder. All mental illnesses are put into groups for easier diagnosis. These groups are called clusters. Cluster A personality is characterised by odd, eccentric thinking or behaviour. You would expect to see schizoid personality disorder and schizotypical personality in Cluster A. Cluster C is characterised by anxious, fearful thinking and behaviour. You would expect to see obsessive personality disorder in Cluster C.

The cluster that we are concerned with here is Cluster B. The main players are:

Histrionic Personality Disorder. HPD. As the words imply, this person is dramatic, erratic and volatile. They become distressed if they are not the centre of attention. You know it when these people are around because they're emotional, expressive and aggressive to the point of embarrassment.

Borderline Personality Disorder. BPD. The person with this condition is emotionally unstable. You do not know what you are going to get on the day. They are impulsive and reckless. Their behaviour is often disruptive and their anger can be terrifying.

Anti- Social Personality Disorder. ASPD, commonly referred to as sociopathy. If you are dealing with a sociopath then you will know it because the sociopath is prone to violence, crime, drugs and has no regard for authority whatsoever. They are aggressive to people, animals and property.

Narcissist Personality Disorder. NPD. Narcissists are disordered. They do not see life the way you and I do. Everything that you believe in, they believe in the complete opposite. They are a mess pretending to be the best.

It is best to think of Cluster B as a family. In any family you can see that the members have individual personalities yet at the same time can see the family resemblance and family traits. This is true for the members of Cluster B. They are different but they like to wear each other's clothes.

All the members in Cluster B are narcissists. It's just that they exhibit narcissism in different ways. All members of Cluster B are grandiose. It is wrong to think that grandiosity is a category of narcissism. Grandiosity is a characteristic of all those in Cluster B. All members of Cluster B do damage to everyone they come across and in that sense they are all anti-social. The Cluster B family is like a box of chocolates: you never know what you are going to get.

Here are some more traits and features that you will get in all of the Cluster B family.

- The Cluster B family are terrorists. Their whole motivation is to conduct a hostile takeover of your mind.

- The Cluster B family are predators who survive by preying on other people.

- The Cluster B family are vampires. They will suck out every last drop of emotion that you have.

- The Cluster B family are zombies. They are the living dead.

- The Cluster B family are chameleons. Like a chameleon they can chop and change to fit in any environment they find themselves in. They watch and wait to pounce on any unsuspecting prey that they identify as food.

- The Cluster B family are assassins. The whole idea is to wipe you out.

- The Cluster B family are parasites. They seek to worm themselves into your brain and live off your emotions. They take your money, live rent free and have you running around like a slave as if it is their right.

Narcissistic behaviour

The Mayo Clinic, The Medical Centre for Health Care, Education and Research say these are the symptoms you will find in a narcissist.

1)   Have an exaggerated sense of self-importance.
2)   Have a sense of entitlement and require constant, excessive admiration.
3)   Expect to be recognised as superior even without achievements that warrant it.
4)   Exaggerate achievements and talents.
5)   Be preoccupied with fantasies about success, power, brilliance, beauty or the perfect mate.
6)   Believe they are superior and can only associate with equally special people.
7)   Monopolise conversations and belittle or look down on people they perceive as inferior.
8)   Expect special favours and unquestioning compliance with their expectations.
9)   Take advantage of others to get what they want.
10) Have an inability or unwillingness to recognise the needs and feelings of others.
11) Be envious of others and believe others envy them.
12) Behave in an arrogant or haughty manner, coming across as conceited, boastful and pretentious.

13) Insist on having the best of everything — for instance, the best car, mobile or smart TV even though they have no means to pay for anything.

14) Have a hard time dealing with any type of criticism.

15) Become impatient or angry when they don't receive special treatment.

16) Have significant interpersonal problems and easily feel slighted.

17) React with rage or contempt and try to belittle the other person to make themselves appear superior.

18) Have difficulty regulating emotions and behaviour.

19) Experience major problems dealing with stress and adapting to change.

20) Feel depressed and moody because they fall short of perfection.

21) Have secret feelings of insecurity, shame, vulnerability and humiliation.

If the person you are dealing with exhibits more than five or six of these behaviours then the chances are you are dealing with a narcissist. It doesn't matter if they are a family member, a boss or a romantic partner; a narcissist is a narcissist is a narcissist.

Understanding the narcissist is a very complicated thing to do. There are many layers. So what do we know so far? We know that the narcissist belongs to the Cluster B family and that all the Cluster B family are narcissists. We know that all the

Cluster B family are anti-social by design. We also know that they are a mish mash of each other's behaviours. They belong to the same family, they share a lot of the same traits and yet they have their own distinct approaches to the 'anti-socialness'. I think I have just made up a word.

THe cLiNicaL NarciSSiSt

Now let's look at what defines a narcissist. The DSM is only concerned with the overt narcissist and the covert narcissist. Despite what you have seen on social media, all narcissist behaviours can be described as either overt or covert. Everything else is a variation on a theme.

The overt narcissist is probably the one that everyone refers to when they talk about narcissism. They have all the classic symptoms that I described earlier but more. The overt narcissist's volume is always on high. In the case of the covert narcissist as their name implies they are not so easy to detect. People think coverts are shy. They are not shy; that's just a cover up for their shitty behaviour.

The covert narcissist is a coward. They are passive aggressive and they do things via the back door. They say things and then swear blind they didn't say it. They are negative, critical of everything and judgemental. They use language in such a way that you can never quite call them out on what they say. They use sarcasm. One of the covert narcissist's greatest pleasures is other people's misfortunes. Tell them that so and so has lost their job and watch their face light up with glee.

They are jealous of other people's fortunes and hate to hear when someone is doing well. You can waste a lot of years on a covert. They are particularly dangerous because the abuse is insidious. Many people don't realise that what they have been putting up with for years is actually abusive toxic behaviour.

Sub-clinical Narcissists

A lot of people who study narcissism have taken some of the behaviours I have listed above and come up with their own narcissist theories. There is nothing wrong with that just as long as you know. For example, you might read about the grandiose narcissist. That is not a category of narcissism recognised by the DSM. Don't go looking for a grandiose narcissist because, as I said before, all narcissists are grandiose.

It should be noted that the DSM takes a long time to review mental health issues. It takes a while for people in the field to research and gather the data.

Let take a look at some other narcissist types that have emerged recently. Who knows, if we gather enough data and research on them they may make the cut in later editions of the DSM. For now they remain sub-clinical.

1. The somatic narcissist can be seen all over social media. They get their supply from the

adoration of millions of followers. They are obsessed with the body beautiful. They have extreme surgeries and blatantly lie about it. They gaslight their followers and feed off their low self-esteem.

2. Then we have the communal narcissist. They are like Jekyll and Hyde. They usually have high status in the community. They can be found in the church, running a football club or involved in a charity group. To the outside world they are humanity personified but in the home behind closed doors the communal narcissist is a monster. They terrorise their family. They beat their children up. Their rages are epic. If you were raised by a communal narcissist then you know all about it. The family suffers in silence. It's the family secret. If you told anyone no one would believe you.

3. Then there is malignant narcissist. The most dangerous narcissist of all. Some say that the malignant narcissist is the hate child of a narcissist and a psychopath. The malignant narcissist is distinguishable by their propensity towards sadism and violence. Sometimes the malignant narcissist is referred to as the Dark Triad, simply because they are evil as hell.

In order to understand the malignant narcissist, I have to tell you about the psychopath. If we are fascinated by the narcissist, we are even more fascinated by the psychopath. We love to see the cold calculated psychopath in action. How far will they go? How evil can they be? How could anyone be that evil? We love to frighten ourselves to death with the idea of the psychopathic serial killer who lives next door. We toy with the idea of outwitting them.

Contrary to popular opinion or what Netflix would have us believe, not all psychopaths are serial killers. Only 1% of the world's population fits the description of a psychopath and only 1% of that 1% ends up as serial killers. People are not born killing machines. There are a lot of things that have to happen before a person takes to killing.

We need psychopaths. If you were off on holiday and your plane ran into heavy turbulence, you would want a cool-headed psychopath as the pilot. If you were going in for surgery you would want a cool, calculating surgeon to operate on you. Maybe the surgeon has no bedside manner, but who cares. They know exactly what they are doing and where to insert the knife. More than that you need someone who wouldn't go into cardiac arrest if you went into cardiac arrest.

We need a James Bond type who will not only fly the plane but get out on the wing of the plane to fight the bad guys. Psychopaths have no fear. They are not bothered by the things that seem to bother the rest of us. The psychopath is James Bond, Jack Reacher and John Wick, all the superheroes that we know and love and all the Marvel characters have psychopathic tendencies. We love to watch them kick the baddie's arse.

We thrill at their daredevil nature, their calmness under fire and their ability to take risks. The psychopath makes good viewing. It isn't so thrilling when the psychopath is your own father, your partner or your boss.

Here is a question that is typically asked by specialists to determine if someone is a psychopath. Not many psychopaths sign up to answer this question so the research is usually taken from psychopaths in jail.

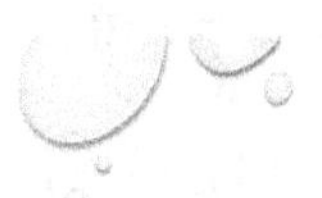

WHO'S THE PSYCHOPATH?

IMAGINE A RUNAWAY TRAIN. IT IS CAREERING TOWARDS SOME UNSUSPECTING CHILDREN PLAYING ON THE TRACK. ON ANOTHER TRACK IS A WORKMAN. IF YOU PULL THE LEVER THE TRAIN WILL BE DIVERTED ON TO THE OTHER TRACK. THE WORKMAN WILL BE KILLED BUT THE CHILDREN WILL BE SAVED. WHAT DO YOU DO?

It's a dilemma for the majority of us but not for the psychopath. They would have no compunction in pulling the lever either way. Killing children or killing a workman is all the same to the psychopath. The psychopath does not do anything because it looks good, they have their own moral compass. They do the right thing for them and if it coincides with the norms of society, then all well and good.

The psychopath has a dotted line to the Cluster B family. They share a lot of similarities in behaviour or so it seems. The main reason why they are not a full member of the Cluster B family is the common belief among the experts that psychopaths are born and all the other personality disorders in the Cluster B family are made. That is to say that the psychopath is spawned from nature and other disorders are spawned from nurture. Psychopaths have different brain wiring to the rest of us.

To understand the mind of a psychopath we have to look at a hormone called serotonin. Serotonin is a chemical produced in the brain and the body that affects the way you feel. It is also responsible for memory, regulating sleep regulations and sexual behaviour and influences the capacity to learn as well. It is well documented that the lack of serotonin is responsible for anxiety and depression. Let's look at serotonin a little closer.

At the end of every synapse in the brain is a space which connects it to another synapse. This space is called the synaptic cleft. The cleft exists so that the wonders of chemistry can take place. The serotonin is released by one neuron and reabsorbed by another. This process is called reuptake. For some reason not all the serotonin leaves the synaptic cleft. It must leave the cleft so that the synapses know exactly how much serotonin is needed for the brain and body to function at any time. The brain breaks down the remaining serotonin by producing an enzyme called monoamine, known as MAOA. What researchers have discovered is that psychopaths have the low functioning variant of MAOA compared to what you would see in people classified as normal. Since psychopaths' brains cannot break down serotonin efficiently, they develop too much serotonin.

But wait, isn't serotonin supposed to be the happy hormone, I hear you say? How can too much serotonin be a bad thing? Well apparently it is. Researchers have found that too much serotonin is linked to aggression.

The fact that someone's brain is unable to break down serotonin effectively because they have low MAOA does not automatically make them a psychopath. So what else is going on?

Patients who displayed symptoms of psychopathy underwent a PET scan and were asked ethical and moral questions, like the one I asked you earlier about the children on the railway line. What researchers found was that when asked a moral dilemma the psychopath had low activity in the prefrontal cortex. So let's say they were told a story of how a child had witnessed their beloved dog get run over by a car. Most of us would show some empathy and there would be high activity in the prefrontal cortex. In the case of the psychopath there was little to no activity whatsoever.

So what do we know so far? We know that psychopaths have low MAOA and so their brain isn't able to break down serotonin efficiently. They are prone to aggression. We also know that they have a defect in the prefrontal cortex which means they are unable to feel empathy. They just don't get empathy. The unique human ability to put yourself in someone else's shoes is anathema to the psychopath.

Even a lack of empathy doesn't make a person a psychopath. There are plenty of people on the planet who do not show empathy and it doesn't make them psychopaths.

Even though a person is born with a brain wired differently to ours we have seen they can still be a valuable member of society. So what is it that makes a person with psychopathic brain wiring turn evil? If you observed a psychopath and a narcissist you wouldn't be able to tell who's who. They share similar traits. They are both narcissists. They are both anti-social. The psychopath has a brain defect that gives them a propensity towards psychopathy but that isn't enough to make them evil. On the contrary, it make them very useful to society. So what is it that goes wrong that turns a psychopath with potential into a psychopath with poison?

I am going to describe the childhood of a few infamous psychopaths that you may have heard of. Tell me what they have in common.

Jeffrey Dahmer was raised in a seemingly good family. Behind the scenes his parents were constantly fighting. His father was a chemist and he had access to chemicals that he would use to dissolve the bodies of dead animals. Dahmer was bullied at school and had no friends. He was a loner. He became an alcoholic in high school. His mother had her own mental issues and when his father moved out she preferred Jeffrey stay alone in the house than go and stay with his father. It was whilst Jeffrey was alone that he killed for the first time.

John Wayne Gacy's father was an alcoholic and often abused his children. John tells a story of being beaten so badly by his father that he was knocked out. He later experienced blackouts and when he did his father would ridicule him and call him a 'sissy'. John Wayne Gacy became "Pogo the Clown". He told people that he wanted to give children the gift of happiness that he didn't get as a child. What he actually gave children was the misery and torture that he had received as a child.

Andrei Chikatilo was a Soviet serial killer. He was born into abject poverty in Stalin's rule. His family would often eat grass to fill their bellies. When Chikatilo was four years old his brother disappeared. His mother took to telling him that his brother had been kidnapped by neighbours and eaten. She terrorised him. Chikatilo kidnapped, tortured, murdered and mutilated the bodies of his victims. Sometimes he would eat the genitalia of his victims or sell their body parts as exotic meat. Charming!

All of these three psychopaths have childhood terror and abuse in common and it is believed that childhood experiences make a psychopath a potential stone cold killer or abuser.

Break

We now know that what makes a psychopath a cold-hearted killer is childhood trauma and child abuse. All the psychopaths whom psychologists have studied over the years and across the globe share this fact.

It is a cliché to say that those that have been abused go on to abuse, but there it is. It seems to be true in the case of the evil psychopath.

As far as we know a narcissist is born with a perfectly normal brain. They have the capacity to develop empathy just like any other person so why do differences emerge?

Now there many schools of thought when it comes to how the narcissist is made. I'll give you two. The first theory states that if a child is overindulged, they will become a narcissist. Well that may be the case but it doesn't really hold up to scrutiny. If a child got everything they wanted, it might make them entitled and arrogant but why would it cause them to ruin other people's lives?

Psychologist Donald Winnicott wasn't buying it either. He said 'A child needs hate to hate'. A narcissist cannot develop out of a kind, warm, loving and well-adjusted family.

There has to be more to narcissism than meets the eye. The second theory is fantastical but probably more likely. According to Sigmund Freud every one of us goes through a narcissist stage in our formative years. This is called the Primary Narcissist Stage. If you make it through this stage intact then you have every chance of winding up a well-adjusted human being with lots of empathy balanced with a healthy sense of self.

Children develop fast. At the same time as the child is going through the Primary Narcissist Stage of child development they also develop magical thinking. You only have to look at a child's face when they are listening to a story to know that they are not only listening to the story, they are 'in' the story living the story chapter by chapter. Children love superheroes. They love to dress up like their favourite superhero. They love acting out stories of superheroes.

Hannah is seven years old. She is going through the Primary Narcissist Stage of child development. She is getting a sense of who she is and with the support and encouragement from her parents she is developing her self-esteem. At the same time as developing a healthy self-esteem Hannah is also in her magical thinking stage where she identifies with a superheroes. Hannah will leave the narcissist and magical stage with a healthy self-esteem, emotional intelligence and the idea that everything is possible.

Sid is also seven years of age and he is also going through the Primary Narcissist Stage and magical thinking stage of child development. But Sid's experiences in this stage are quite different from Hannah's. Sid is being abused. He is being attacked by those whom he loves and those who should love him. All Sid receives is criticism, blame and judgement and so he has no means with which to develop self-esteem. If he isn't shown kindness and encouragement during this stage of his development then he has no means with which to develop empathy and consideration for others. In Sid's mind he has to survive the onslaught of attack. It's a matter of life and death. Sid disconnects from reality and goes off to a fantasy world where he himself is the superhero.

Do you see the difference here? Hannah identifies with the superhero but she and her superhero are quite separate entities. Sid on the other hand fuses with the superhero and cannot be separated. Sid becomes the superhero as a matter of survival.

Sid lives in a fantasy land of his own making. What's the worst that could happen? The worst thing that could happen actually happens to Sid. He cannot give up his fantasy land because that would mean he would have to suffer the pain of the abuse that sends him to his fantasy land in the first place. So he is stuck. While his peers are developing self-esteem, interpersonal skills and emotional intelligence, Sid is still playing heroes and villains. Sid is always the hero. Everyone is either a hero or a villain. All villains must be destroyed at any cost. That is the black or white thinking of a superhero and that is the black or white thinking of a narcissist.

There are problems in Sid's fantasy land. Number 1: Sid cannot come down from fantasy land because in his mind he would have to suffer the abuse that sent him to fantasy land in the first place. Number 2: basking in the sunshine of your own amazingness is fun sometimes but boring most of the time. Narcissists need entertaining. Number 3: no one helped Sid develop self-esteem and so his ideas around self-esteem and feeling good about himself is warped. He is empty inside. He has no self. He has no emotions. He needs people to feed him with emotions and adoration in order for him to know he exists. Number 4: it is lonely on

Fantasy Island. A narcissist has to hatch a cunning plan to get you to join them on Fantasy Island.

It is very simple. The narcissist tells you that they are amazing. They then tell you that you too are amazing and they cannot live without you. You feel amazing because someone so amazing has fallen in love with you. They whisk you off to Fantasy Island to fatten you up with stories of how amazing you both are together.

The minute you question paradise you fall from grace and you become the villain that must be destroyed.

This seems like a good place to stop. Tomorrow we will see how a narcissist goes about destroying people.

What questions do you have at this point?"

"Can a narcissist change"?

"There are many ways to answer this question. Yes of course the narcissist can change. As I told you before, they are chameleons. They can adapt to any situation to get what they want. No of course they cannot change. Narcissism is a personality disorder. This disorder means that they don't have the capacity to change and even if they did what would they change into? They have no self-awareness so how could they change? Furthermore as far as the narcissist is concerned they are perfect. So why would you change if you believe that you are perfection?

I have a question for you: why should you care if the narcissist can change or not? Are you asking because you think that you are the one that they will change for? Are you asking because you want to play the martyr and sacrifice your own mental health for the benefit of the narcissist? You cannot even love them into changing. You cannot love someone out of psychopathy. You cannot love a narcissist into loving you. You cannot love a narcissist into loving themselves".

"Can a narcissist recognise what they have done and say sorry"?

"That is typical of a narcissist. A narcissist will never simply say 'I'm sorry, I was wrong'. They have to tell you why they did it. What made them do it and who was to blame for them doing it. One of the hallmarks of a narcissist is that they cannot say sorry. Let me qualify that assertion. A narcissist can say sorry but they have no idea what saying sorry means. In order to say sorry you have to have self-awareness and understand that what you did upset somebody. You cannot do this if you have no empathy. The narcissist has no empathy. They can feign empathy but they do this to get themselves off the hook".

"Could a narcissist change by getting therapy?"

"The short answer is 'no'. Oh and a narcissist will never go to therapy unless it suits them. For example, if the narcissist has gone too far, they may say that they will go to therapy just to buy some time. They might indulge in therapy so they can use psychobabble to hook prospective supply. They might even enjoy therapy. Where else can you speak solely about yourself for an hour? In the end the narcissist will get nothing out of therapy because in their mind you cannot improve on perfection".

"What happens when you tell a narcissist that they are a narcissist?"

"Why would you do that? To tell someone that they are a narcissist without any clinical qualification is actually what a narcissist would do. What is your intention behind telling them that they are a narcissist? Do you think that by telling them that they are a narcissist that they will thank you? Do you think that by you telling them what they are they will wake up and see the error of their ways and be indebted to you forever? When you tell a narcissist that they are a narcissist you put a big target on your head. You have committed the worst sin of all. You criticised a narcissist. You have identified yourself as an enemy. All bets are off and the narcissist's gloves are put on. They will turn up the abuse because you need to be punished for calling them out. If they can't be bothered to punish you they will simply ghost you and block you".

"Can a relationship with a narcissist work?"

"Of course a relationship can work. It depends what you mean by 'work'. A relationship with a narcissist will work if you are prepared to live your live in sacrifice to a complete arsehole.

Ok everyone, let's wrap up for today. Go and have your treatments and take advantage of as much of the facilities as you can.

See you tomorrow. Have a good evening"!

TUESDAY

- THE STORY OF NARCISSUS
- THE CYCLE OF ABUSE
- THE TRAUMA BOND
- CHILDREN OF THE NARCISSIST PARENT

"Good morning all. I trust you all slept well"?

They nodded.

"I hope you all managed to take advantage of the treatments and facilities".

They nodded again.

"I must say, you are all positively glowing!"

All of them had managed to get a treatment. They compared notes. The cranial massage was top of the leaderboard so far.

"Yesterday, what did we do? Well we defined the narcissist. It is important to note that narcissism is not a mental illness, it is a personality disorder. The DSM, the reference book for all psychiatrists and psychologists in the field, places narcissism in a category called Cluster B. Cluster B houses all those who exhibit anti-social personality disorders. Today we are going to examine in some detail the narcissist, the cycle of abuse and their weapons of choice.

Before we do that we need to understand where the idea of the narcissist comes from.

Let's start at the very beginning.

The Story of Narcissus

The word 'narcissist' comes from Greek mythology. It's a cautionary tale about what happens when you are too vain. There are many versions of the story. I will tell you a couple and you can decide which one you prefer.

Version one. It is said that Narcissus was a very beautiful boy and by the time he was sixteen years old he had many suitors. He didn't look at any of them because as far as he was concerned there was no one to match his beauty. One day as he stopped to drink from the river, he caught sight of his own reflection in the water and immediately fell in love. Despite everyone telling him to leave the river, he didn't. He stayed and pined away. His grieving family went off to get something to transport the body back to the village but when they came back Narcissus's body was nowhere to be seen. All that remained in the place where Narcissus had perished was a single yellow flower. They called the flower narcissus after him. In this version Narcissus dies because he was vain and stupid.

Version two is a little more sinister. It is said that the Gods spoke to Narcissus's mother and told her that Narcissus would live to a ripe old age if he didn't recognise himself. The mother got rid of all the mirrors in the house so he couldn't see himself. Just as in version one of the tale, Narcissus had many suitors including a boy called Ameinias. It is said that Narcissus was outraged and disgusted by the boy and tormented him mercilessly. He eventually gave Ameinias a sword and told him to kill himself. Ameinias finally killed himself outside Narcissus's house but before he died he begged the Gods to curse Narcissus. In this version Echo also falls hopelessly in love with Narcissus. She follows him around everywhere, desperately trying to get him to love her. He shuns her and she finally pines away alone in the forest beside a cave. To this day if you shout in the forest or in a cave, Echo hears you and repeats back to you the last words of what you say. Narcissus got his validation from torturing the people who fell in love with him. One day he saw his own reflection in the river and fell in love with himself. Narcissus got a taste of his own medicine and pined away looking at himself.

In the Greek myth Narcissus has no self-awareness and the only way that he knows he's beautiful is by the amount of people who fawn over him. The narcissist has no self-awareness. They literally cannot recognise themselves. They have no idea who they are. It is common to believe that the narcissist is full of themselves but they are not. They are empty inside.

The narcissist has none of the emotions you and I would class as positive. They have no idea what empathy, kindness and love are; they see that these emotions are important to people; so they feign them. Narcissists are actors. In fact they are Oscar award-winning actors.

They can act out an emotion but they cannot feel emotions. So they do the next best thing. They steal emotions. They don't understand emotions or how they work. They don't know the difference between positive and negative emotions. To a narcissist an emotion is an emotion. As long as they get a reaction out of their victim then they feel important.

By the way, in the world of narcissism the victim is called the 'supply'.

THe NarcissiStic CycLe oF AbuSe

Let's talk about the narcissistic cycle of abuse.

A plumber uses a monkey wrench to fix a leak. I want you to understand that the narcissist is not separate from the cycle of abuse like a plumber is separate from their monkey wrench. The narcissistic cycle of abuse is not a tool. The narcissist is the cycle of abuse and the cycle of abuse is the narcissist. There is no separation. Once you are caught up in this cycle, you will go around and around it like a piece of rag in a tumble dryer. You are being emotionally rinsed.

I am now going to go through the narcissistic cycle of abuse. As I go through it, make a mental note what stage of the cycle you think you are on. It will not be too hard to know. It will be obvious to you. Narcissists are never subtle.

There are three main stages of the narcissistic cycle of abuse.

The first stage of the cycle is the idealisation stage, commonly referred to as love bombing. The next stage is called devaluation and this is often referred to as gaslighting. The final stage is the discarding stage. This is the stage where the narcissist throws you out like the trash when they think that there is nothing left to extract from you.

It doesn't matter who you are and what your relationship is with the narcissist, you will go through this cycle in varying degrees of intensity and duration. What you have to understand is that it doesn't matter what your relationship with the narcissist is, they only have one string to their bow and that is the cycle of abuse. The narcissist doesn't care whether you are their child, mother, father, sister, brother, friend or boss, the narcissist is only in it for supply. I am repeating myself because this is the most important thing for you to understand. The narcissist doesn't care who you are to them. As far as the narcissist is concerned supply is thicker than blood.

Idealisation

The narcissist sees you and hones in on you. There is something about you. Many think that the narcissist chooses people because they are weak. I beg to differ. Others say that the narcissist loves to choose people that are empaths. Maybe empaths are easy targets simply because we take people at face value and give people the benefit of the doubt. Actually it's not that deep. The narcissist chooses anyone in their path. If a narcissist is in need of supply they will choose anyone. Even if they do not need supply they may line up supply for later. Narcissists get bored very easily. So they may play with potential supply just for the fun of it.

The workings of a narcissist have nothing to do with love and everything to do with supply. Do not take it personally. Supply to a narcissist is people's emotions. If they can control people's emotions then that is as close as they can get to being human and to feeling anything.

The problem is that the narcissist can't tell the difference between the emotions and they don't care. They don't understand happiness or love in the true sense of the words. Oh, they can feign emotions but it doesn't seem the same, it doesn't give them any satisfaction and it never lasts. This is because the narcissist is empty inside. Love is a feeling. The narcissist doesn't have the capacity to feel love. I repeat, the narcissist is empty inside. You cannot grow emotions where no emotions exist. The narcissist's capacity to feel was cauterised in childhood.

Like a vampire that constantly needs blood in order to survive, the narcissist needs emotions in order to survive.

The narcissist chooses a supply. They choose a supply depending on what they need. Perhaps they need money or a place to stay. Maybe they need a slave. Someone who will wash, cook, clean, iron, fetch and carry for them. Or maybe they need someone to ferry them around. Maybe you have status in your job or the community and they want to bask in your glory and then steal your glory. Narcissists also choose supply based on what they are into. Narcissists need supply to pay for their predilections. Sex, porn, gambling, drugs and buying shiny new stuff.

According to Professor of Psychology Sam Vaknim, the narcissist takes a photo of you in their head and then 'photoshops' you. The photo that they take of you in their mind is perfect. By the way, the photo they take of you has nothing to do with you and may not even look like you. They need supply and you happen to be there. Now the whole idea is to get you to fall for them and the way they achieve this is to make out as if they have fallen for you. They shower you with attention and affection like nothing you have experienced before. When a narcissist sets their sights on you it is very difficult to resist their charm.

If it's going to take months to get you hooked then they will pursue you until they get you hooked. They will bombard you with texts. First thing in the morning and last thing at night. They send you a text just to say that they are thinking of you. They send you another to ask if you have eaten. If it is cold outside they tell you wrap up warm.

In the beginning the relationship is intense. You have never been cared for like this before. One of the ways that a narcissist gets under your skin is to find areas in your life where you feel dissatisfaction. It doesn't matter what it is, they will keep digging until they find it.

You being the innocent fresh supply may think that the narcissist is asking questions because they are enamoured by you. No! That isn't the case. The narcissist digs until they find your weak points, your issues, your vulnerabilities and your insecurities. They gather everything on you to use against you later and you will not be able to say a thing because it was you yourself that fed them the information with which they will destroy you at a later date.

Let me show you how a narcissist works.

Let's say you are at an event, enjoying yourself and minding your own business. By the way a narcissist hates human gatherings. They don't get them. They don't understand why people want to get together, to chat, celebrate and enjoy each other's company without any strings attached.

The narcissist attends events for one reason only and that is to set up fresh supply. Even though they hate events they know how to play the game. Narcissists are expert at networking. They can work a room adeptly, talking to people and telling jokes. Making people fall in love with them. They use the adoration of an audience to get a few nibbles of supply. Like an appetiser. All the while they are on the lookout for the main meal.

When you meet someone at an event, the conversation will go something like this:

"Hello my name is X and you are?"

"Hello, pleased to meet you my name is Bev".

"What do you do Bev"?

"I work with people".

"Oh that's great".

In this scenario, two people meet, have a brief exchange, and decide whether they have anything in common. They decide to talk more or to make an excuse and move on.

If you are talking to a narcissist and that narcissist is hungry for supply you are not going to get away so easily. Your conversation will go something like this:

"Hello my name is Narc and you are?"

"I'm Bev."

"Wow! Bev that is a lovely name. My grandmother was called 'Bev'. We were really close. Bev you look amazing! Perhaps I shouldn't say this, but your dress shows off your beautiful body. I didn't want to come tonight, but I am so glad I did. You have made my night".

Right there, can you see the narcissist's game? First they compliment you. Then they tell you that someone who means a lot to them has something in common with you. The conversation will move from introductions to something intimate very quickly. All the time they are testing you to see how far they can go with you, if you have any boundaries and if so what they are. The will suss out what kind of supply you will make. You could be the main line, a side line or you could be an emergency lifeline set up for later. And you, you don't notice a thing. As far as you are concerned you are having an exhilarating, heady and edgy conversation, your body flooded with the hormone oxytocin. You feel connected and alive. You are being groomed and you are loving it.

A narcissist may hook you by telling you how amazing, beautiful or funny you are; and you lap it up. They will tell you anything that they think you want to hear. Despite all their failings as human beings, narcissists are really good at reading people.

Here is an example of a conversation with a normal person.

"What do you do"?

"I am a nuclear physicist".

"Oh that's sounds exciting..."

Here is an example of a conversation with a narcissist.

"What do you do"?

"I am a nuclear physicist".

"So tell me does your job fulfil you"?

"Well not really...how could you tell"?

"Because I can feel we have a connection".

"My boss doesn't appreciate me".

"It so frustrating when people don't appreciate you. I appreciate you Bev. I appreciate someone as smart as you talking to me. I appreciate your smile. What's the matter with your boss? They are mad. How could anyone not appreciate you?"

Boom! You're hooked. The narcissist asks you about your frustrations, concerns, dissatisfactions and then they set out to be the answer to your prayers. If you feel misunderstood they understand you. If you are lonely they will become your trusty companion. Whatever you need in your life the narcissist is the answer. They make themselves the answer.

The next part of the 'plan' is to get you to adore them. They have to get you to fall head over heels in love with them. The way that they do this is to tell you that they have fallen in love with you. It's the oldest trick in the book.

This process of you falling in love with them is called the Idealisation Stage or **love bombing**. During the love bombing stage, they tell you:

"You are so easy to talk to..."

"I feel I can tell you anything..."

"I have never opened up to anyone like this before..."

"I see my future with someone like you..."

"With you by my side I feel as if I could do anything."

"I need you in my life."

The narcissist goes from hello to intimacy in no time at all. They are fast and furious. A narcissist uses sex to get you loved up. They will have you swinging from the chandeliers, seeing stars and singing 'arias' you never knew you could sing. You have a lot of sex. They make sure of it. The sex is addictive. You feel special. You get addicted to the idea of love. You get addicted to them. You get addicted to the way they make you feel.

You can't believe that this amazing person is in love with you. You are now well and truly in the love bombing stage. Everything that you ever fantasied about how true love should be is what the narcissist gives you. Your life is just like the movies.

Narcissists do this thing called **future faking**. In the love bombing stage they will build a future of the two of you together. They ask you about your dreams for the future, you innocently tell them and lo and behold their dreams are the same as yours. If you want ten children, they want ten children. If you dream of travelling the world they dream of travelling the world. Fancy that! What are the chances of meeting someone who shares the same dreams as you? It must be destiny. It isn't destiny, it's faking the future and what's more it is never going to happen. The whole idea of future faking is for you to feel safe, secure and to drop your guard.

The narcissist has to get under your skin. They do it by using reciprocity. I'll tell you my secrets if you tell me yours. You pour your heart out and they lie through their teeth.

They tell you something about themselves. They also tell you that they have never told anybody their secret before. You feel privileged and all loved up. You drop your guard and tell them everything. Your hopes, fears, vulnerability and insecurities. You think that is making your connection stronger. Wrong. Little do you know that they are building a dossier on you, to use against you and to destroy you when the time comes. They will make you out to be a hypocrite if you do anything that contradicts with anything you have told them about yourself in the past. What's more you will never be able to challenge them about anything they do because they will throw it back in your face.

'I told you everything there is to know about me... so you can't complain that you didn't know'.

Those are the kind of remarks that leave you flabbergasted. There is no way you can argue with a narcissist unless you enjoy arguing with a four year old. They will tie you up in a word soup so that eventually you will be the one agreeing with them just to shut them up.

As I said, the narcissist has to get you hooked on love very quickly. The relationship is like a whirlwind. They cannot afford to allow you to catch your breath. A narcissist declares undying love within days not months or years. Now the reason why they have to move in on you so quickly is to distract you, so that you do not get time to notice their disordered behaviour or the red flags waving right under your nose.

If you were to pause for a moment you could notice the following things: their stories don't add up, they talk about their exes in a disparaging way and they are rude to people. They lose their temper at the slightest provocation. They sulk when they don't get what they want. They do not have any friends. They love it when others fail. They are estranged from their family. They have big plans but never seem to put in any effort. They are never wrong. They spent a lot of time gaming, sleeping, on the mobile, watching porn. They drink and probably take drugs. They are opinionated. They are rigid in their thinking. They have selective memory and they only remember things that suit their narrative. They have no sense of humour. They are easily bored. As for lying, narcissists are compulsive liars. Even when you are with them you never feel as if you are with them. They walk in front of you or behind. They disappear in a crowd so that you spend your time trying to track them down.

I could go on and on. I am sure you could add a lot more to this list.

Devaluation

At some point, as sure as day follows night, you are going to fall from grace. Not because there is anything wrong with you. No! You fall from grace because you start to see the narcissist for who they are. Despite all the big talk nothing makes sense. They talk about money but they never have any. They talk about all the people who adore them but they have no friends. They talk about big plans for the future but they don't seem to have any follow-through. None of their plans ever get off the ground. Nothing is ever their fault. The narcissist never takes responsibility for anything and their excuses are flimsy. You realise that the narcissist is flawed and you start to offer advice, but the narcissist being who they are sees your advice as criticism. The narcissist cannot be criticised in any form or fashion. Criticism is the narcissist's kryptonite. They are super sensitive to it. When you criticise a narcissist, even with good intentions, it is the kiss of death for the relationship and in the eyes of a narcissist, you must be punished for daring to see them as anything other than perfect.

Gaslighting is one of the best known terms used when describing narcissistic behaviour. Most people use the term gaslighting as shorthand to describe behaviour they don't like. Gaslighting is much more than that. Only those who have been exposed to the full extent of gaslighting understand the full meaning of the term. The verb gaslight comes from the 1938 play and the

1944 film adaptation 'Gaslight'. The story is about a man who marries for money. In order to get his hands on his wife's inheritance he has to get her to doubt her own reality and convince her that she is mad. In one famous scene he tampers with the lights above the apartment where he and his wife live, causing them to dim and flicker. When his wife tells him that the lights dim and flicker, he tells her that she is imagining things. Getting you to doubt your own take on reality is the main feature of gaslighting.

Gaslighting may start in an innocuous way. They may move things around and pretend they didn't move it. They may say something and swear blind they never said it. They will hide things and watch you tear your hair out trying to find it.

If you question a narcissist on their behaviour, here are some of the typical responses you will get:

"You're crazy that's not what happened."

"This is all your fault, I don't know why I listen to you."

"Look what happened, you are such a waste of space."

"You are useless. I don't know why I put up with you."

Once they have embarked on devaluing you their onslaught is relentless. They distort your words. Make fun of your tears, delete information that doesn't suit their narrative and distort the facts to suit them.

If you try to challenge their behaviour, here are some of the typical responses you will get:

"It's not that big a deal, get over it."

"You are overthinking this."

"I was only joking when I called you a fucking idiot. Where's your sense of humour these days."

"You are so emotional it's really hard work talking to you."

Gaslighting gets you to doubt your own sanity and your sense of reality. It destabilises you. The narcissist weakens your sense of self to the point where you don't know whether you are coming or going or whether your name is Martha or Arthur. You get your emotional cues from the narcissist. If they are happy then you can relax. It becomes your sole purpose to make them happy. If they are unhappy then you feel inadequate and responsible.

I feel I need to clarify something here. Yesterday I said that the narcissist by definition is disordered. Today I am talking about the narcissistic cycle of abuse. This suggests that the narcissist has a system. I don't want you to go away thinking that the narcissist has a system. It might seem like it but they don't. They work on instinct. Like a lizard. If they need supply they will do whatever they need to do and say whatever they need to say to get what they want. Abuse is not something a narcissist does abuse is what the narcissist is.

Break

Even before the devaluation stage the narcissist will set about isolating you from your friends and family. It is what they do. It may appear innocent at first. They may say:

"I want to be with you every hour of the day."

"If we have each other we don't need anyone else".

Then it escalates to this:

"Why do you have to speak to your mother every day"?

So now you begin to feel self-conscious about speaking to your own mother. They don't like it. You don't want to cause a scene. So you stop calling your mother. The narcissist doesn't stop until they have isolated you from everyone.

All of a sudden the narcissist never wants to go to any event organised by your friends and family. If they go they sulk. You have to make excuses for them all the time. You 'dumb' down on your behaviour because if they so much as get a whiff that you are having a good time you will pay later. You stop attending family events or going out with your friends. Your hobbies, pastimes and interests that you used to enjoy become things of the past. Eventually family and friends stop inviting you and they drift away. The narcissist wants this because they do not want you to have a support system or anyone coming to your defence when they abuse you. They want you isolated and alone so that they can feast on you with impunity.

One of the ways that the narcissist punishes you for your 'bad behaviour' is by sulking. I do not know what the record is for sulking, but narcissists can sulk for days, months or even years. When a narcissist sulks they give you the silent treatment and in narcissistic circles this is called is called **stonewalling**. You will get stonewalled if the narcissist perceives that you have done something wrong. The thing is that you may not even be aware that you have done something wrong and the narcissist isn't going to tell you what you did wrong because they are stonewalling you. The narcissist gets up one day and decides to stonewall you. When you are being stonewalled, as far as the narcissist is concerned you don't exist. If you speak to them they will answer only if they have to. They will not acknowledge your presence. If you try to start a conversation they will not hide their irritation. Rolling their eyes and tutting. Stonewalling makes you feel like shit. It has you walking around on eggshells in your own home. Not knowing if you are coming or going. You may find yourself apologising like a peasant to the sire for something you didn't even do. In fact you may find yourself apologising for something that they did.

Yes, the narcissist isolates you from your friends and family but they are not averse to using your friends and family against you. Let me show you how it works in this example.

Let's say you and the narcissist have fallen out. It is their fault. Any normal person would apologise. The narcissist cannot apologise.

They do not have the mechanism with which to do so. As I said before, in order to apologise you have to care that you have hurt someone. Instead of taking responsibility for their actions the narcissist uses **triangulation**. The narcissist sends in your friend to do their dirty work for them and to mess with your emotions.

Your friend will say things like this:

"They only acted that way because they love you, haven't been sleeping well lately, lost their job, got a speeding ticket". You name it, it could be anything.

Triangulation puts you in a dilemma. Do you listen to your friend who you know and trust or do you listen to your gut? Triangulation is a form of manipulation designed to get you to question your own moral standards and values. You lose sight of the fact that they behaved badly and start to feel sorry for them. You then feel guilty for calling them out on their bad behaviour. Again you are the one that ends up apologising. If the narcissist successfully breaks down your morals and values then they can replace them with their own fucked up ones.

Another way that the narcissist uses your friends and family against you is by recruiting them to do their bidding. The narcissist sets this up with your nearest and dearest by telling them that they are concerned about you and that they need to watch you. The narcissist recruits **flying monkeys** to spy on you. The term flying monkeys was first observed in the film 'The Wizard of Oz'. In the movie the Wicked Witch sent flying monkeys to do her dirty work. The flying monkeys are the narcissist's henchmen. Flying monkeys fall for the narcissist's charm and they want to do right by them. It doesn't matter what your relationship is with the flying monkey, they will throw you under the bus in favour of the narcissist.

Flying monkeys carry out the following assignments for the narcissist:

1. They spy on you and report back. All of a sudden the narcissist knows exactly who you've talked to and where you have been. This is very intimidating.

2. They stalk you and report back. You feel that you are being watched and you are constantly looking over your shoulder. This is very unsettling.

3. They spread gossip and rumours about you. This is bewildering because it seems like everyone has turned against you and you do not know who to trust.

Maya Angelou once said that when people show you who they are you need to believe them. This is particularly true when you are dealing with flying monkeys. Flying monkeys are not your family and neither are they your friends. A Flying monkey is the narcissist's apprentice. A flying monkey is a narcissist in waiting.

DISCARD

At some point the narcissist discards you. It is not a question of if you will be discarded it's a question of when. The narcissist doesn't have to leave your life to discard you. The discard is a psychological act. You could be living in the same house as the narcissist and feel as if you are living with a stranger.

When people go through a break up, as painful as it may be at least both parties know that they are going through a breakup. With a narcissist you have no clue what is going on. One minute you are in a relationship, well at least that's what you thought and the next minute you have been unceremoniously dumped. Suddenly you are persona non grata. You have been kicked to the kerb like something on the bottom of the narcissist shoe. If you are in the discard stage you will know it.

The abuse you will suffer during the discard stage is off the chart. It certainly is verbal and oftentimes it is physical. One of the main features of the discard stage is the narcissistic rage. You have to see this to believe it. Many people who have witnessed the narcissistic rage say that the whole face of the narcissist contorts to the point where their features become unrecognisable. Their eyes literally change colour. When you look into their eyes you see the abyss. There is no one there. In this stage the narcissistic mask slips and you get to see the terrifying cruelty that they are capable of. During the discard stage be prepared for an experience worse than hell.

The narcissist never breaks up with you, they discard you only so that they can hook up with you in the future if they run low on supply. Even though the narcissist tells you that you are nothing they will still keep tabs on you. They watch your social media activities and they check up on you through your friends. Your friends might think that the narcissist is concerned about your wellbeing. Far from it. The narcissist is checking up on you to find out if you have found someone else and then they will come in and mess that up. They check up to see if you have got your act together enough to offer them fresh supply. If they think you have supply they will sweep in and attempt to swoop you up. This activity is called **hoovering.**

I'll tell you how hoovering works. You may have gone 'no contact' and are in the process of getting your life back together when out of the blue you get a text from the narcissist.

They may say something like this:

"I was going through some old photos and came across a photo of us together at the lovely

restaurant we used to go. Would you like to see it?"

• They might text you on your birthday or Christmas.

• They might like something that you posted on social media or suddenly appear in a chat or online.

• They may turn up at an event you are attending or even show up at your place of work.

If the narcissist targets you for hoovering you will not be able to make a move until they feel that you are back under their spell. If you go back to the narcissist after being discarded it is simply because the narcissist is low on supply. If you go back, the narcissist is aware of how much abuse you can take and how much you are prepared to put up with. In this way they don't have to mess around with love bombing. They don't even have to pretend to like you. They don't have to pretend to be someone they are not. You have seen them at their worst. If you take a narcissist back after they have discarded you be prepared to be treated like shit.

During the discard stage the narcissist takes off their mask and puts on their gloves. They do not care how they behave in front of you. In fact the more they terrorise you the better they feel. Your distress makes them feel superior.

During the discard stage their behaviour becomes increasingly impulsive and erratic. They make decisions which make no sense. If you challenge them on anything they do they are likely to fly into a rage like you've never seen before. You learn to walk around on eggshells. They become reckless like driving too fast. They take risks like gambling with money they don't have.

During the discard the narcissist seeks to drain the last dregs of supply out of you and so they switch up their behaviour a notch or two. They become downright evil. Their onslaught on you is relentless. It seems as if you have to pay for everything that they hate in the world and narcissists hate a lot. If they speak to you at all it is with utter disgust and contempt.

They may become violent towards you. Lashing out, swearing and shouting, throwing and breaking things.

During the discard stage you will have sex with the narcissist if they cannot get it anywhere else. Sex is transactional. They use sex to reward you, control you, to get what they want out of you and to punish you. Sex is functional. The narcissist uses you just to get the job done. If you complain you will be made to feel dirty, nasty, a sex maniac and debauched.

If you are asking the question 'does a narcissist cheat'. The answer to that is almost certainly yes. Simply because sex to them is transactional and biological. Nothing more nothing less. If the narcissist wants something they have no problem paying with sex.

The trauma bond

Once you have fallen from paradise with the narcissist, you now enter the gates of hell. The narcissist doesn't want you but they will not let you go. One minute you are the best thing since sliced bread the next minute you are something they stepped in. You walk around on eggshells. This creates a perfect storm of chemicals in your system to create what is referred to as the trauma bond. The hormones in question are oxytocin, dopamine, adrenalin and cortisol. Let us see how these hormones work to create a trauma bond.

In the beginning when the narcissist walks into the room you get butterflies and your heart skips a beat. Your body releases adrenalin. It feels wonderful. The way they look at you as if you are the only one that matters. Your body releases oxytocin. You feel proud that you have finally found the one. Your body releases dopamine. Now, when they walk into the room you feel a sense of dread, you do not know what is going to happen next. You release adrenalin but not in a good way. You begin to obsess who they are talking to, who they are with and what they are doing with whoever they are with. You become obsessed with finding out what they are doing. Your body gives you a dose of dopamine, but not in a good way. Every time they speak harshly to you, criticise or treat you like shit you get a rush of cortisol and you become confused. You can't sleep, eat or think straight if they are not around you.

This is a trauma bond. You are addicted. Just like an addict is addicted to heroin, you are addicted to the narcissist. The heroin addict knows that heroin is bad for them but they will do anything for their next hit. You also know that the narcissist is bad for you yet you will do anything to have them around.

This is cognitive dissonance. In short, cognitive dissonance occurs when the brain receives two conflicting pieces of information at the same time. For example, people who smoke know full well that smoking is bad for them. Yet they continue to smoke because smoking makes them feel good and they don't have the resilience to stop. When cognitive dissonance occurs the brain follows the path of least resistance. By the same token you know that the narcissist is bad for you but you don't have the resilience to leave.

I am going to explain a syndrome called the Stockholm Syndrome. Some of you may have heard of it before. It will give you some insight into what actually goes on in a trauma bond.

The Stockholm Syndrome is also known as 'terror bonding' or 'traumatic bonding' and is a paradoxical and psychological phenomenon in which hostages feel empathy and positive feelings toward their captors – sometimes even defending them. Over time, a hostage victim may come to believe that the abuse they have endured was out of kindness or love on the part of the captor.

Back in 1972, two men entered a bank in Stockholm, Sweden, intending to rob it. The police were called, and when they burst into the bank, the two robbers shot them, thus beginning a hostage situation.

For six long days, these robbers held hostage four people who had been in the bank at the time. They were held at gunpoint, sometimes strapping explosives on them and at other times putting nooses around their necks.

The hostages suffered yet by the time the police were able to attempt a rescue, the hostages fought the police off in defence of their captors, blaming the situation entirely upon the police. Once free, one of the hostages set up a fund to cover his captor's legal fees.

The term 'Stockholm Syndrome' was coined to describe the bizarre essence of the captor/ prisoner phenomenon.

The features of Stockholm Syndrome include some of the following:

• Positive feelings from the prisoner toward the captor.

• Negative feelings from the prisoner toward his or her family, friends or authorities attempting any support.

• Support for the captor's reasons and excusing their erratic behaviours.

- Inability by the victim to escape or execute behaviours that suggest that they want to escape or detach from the captor.

In order for Stockholm Syndrome to occur, there must be at least three of the following conditions present:

- There must be a highly uneven balance of power in which the captor must dictate what the captive can and cannot do.

- There must be the threat of death or physical injury to the captive from the captor.

- There must be a self-preservation instinct within the prisoner.

- The prisoner believes (perhaps falsely) that they cannot escape.

- The hostage feels that survival is dependent upon following the rules of the captor.

- The prisoner must be isolated from others who are not being held captive.

Here is a typical example of Stockholm Syndrome.

1. After a very emotionally traumatic and stressful situation, a person finds themselves held captive by a captor who threatens to kill or hurt them if they do not follow the rules. Abuse – physical or emotional or both – occurs. The prisoner has difficulty thinking straight – escape is not an option, right? If they try to escape, something awful may happen.

The prisoner believes that the only way for everyone to survive is to be obedient to the captor.

2. Time marches on. The captor is under stress, and becomes more demanding and erratic. The fluctuating moods of the captor lead to unexpected violence and abuse. The prisoner then learns what triggers may or may not set off their captor as a means of survival.

This, however, means that *the prisoner learns more about his or her captor.*

3. The prisoner begins to see the captor as being kind. Sometimes they may be allowed to try new things, go for a new job or even travel abroad. In this way, the captor plays good cop/ bad cop.

The slightest act of kindness feels like a sign of a connection that the prisoner clings to.

4. Over time, the captor begins to appear less and less threatening and more of a means of survival than harm. In order to survive psychologically and to ease the crisis situation in their life, the prisoner begins to believe that the captor is actually a friend, that they will not kill them and that they can work together to get out of the mess they're in. Rather than see the people on the outside trying to rescue the prisoner as the saviours, instead, they appear to be enemies – they will hurt the captor who is now his or her 'friend' and 'protector.'

The captor has gone from 'captor' to 'friend' in a process of self-delusion and self-preservation on the part of the prisoner.

5. This bonding leads to incredibly conflicted feelings within the prisoner and abuser. The prisoner may begin to feel concern for the captor and at times ignoring their own needs.

6. When the traumatic event is over, the victim can undergo an incredibly hard transition.

The emotional entanglement of Stockholm Syndrome can last a lifetime.

Stockholm Syndrome is a form of traumatic bonding and explains a lot of what happens psychologically in an abusive relationship. In your case, the narcissist is the captor and you are the hostage. Different names, same mess. The only difference is that in a hostage situation the hostage can't leave. They may be tied up or have a gun pointed at their head. In your case there is no gun pointing at you. So why don't they leave? Why don't you pack your bags and leave? Why don't you tell your abuser to 'fuck off' and leave you alone? That is never going to happen.

You see, for a trauma bond to be a trauma bond you have unconsciously identify with your abuser for your survival.

So when the narcissist tells you:

"You are nothing without me".

"If it weren't for me I don't know where you'd be".

"No one's ever gonna want you. You're disgusting!"

"You're gonna to die alone".

"You're useless. Can't you do anything right"?

You believe them.

Break

I want to spend a moment to talk about narcissistic parents. I want you to know before I continue, that the narcissistic cycle of abuse is the same no matter what your relationship with the narcissist is. Narcissists have but one string to their bow and that is the cycle of abuse. As we have seen, if you have a romantic relationship with the narcissist you are going to go through the full cycle of abuse from love bombing to discarding. If you are a child of a narcissist there is no reason on this planet for them to love bomb you. As far as the narcissist parent is concerned, they made you and they already own you.

Children of narcissist parents do not get love bombed. It isn't necessary. You are already a captive audience. They don't have to pretend to even like you. The narcissist cannot relate to humans especially if they are not getting anything from that person. The narcissist parent cannot see the point of children unless the children can do something for them. As far as I can see the only reason narcissists have children is because it's something to do. In fact they end up resenting their own children because children being children are hard work and hard work is something the narcissist can't do. The narcissist sees the world in black or white, good or bad, right or wrong. There are no grey areas as far as the narcissist is concerned. To make the chore of raising children make sense, the narcissist assigns each of their offspring an identity and a role. To the narcissist parent a child is either good, bad, useful or a waste of space.

The Scapegoat Child is the truth teller. They will call the narcissist parent out if they notice inconsistencies and injustice. The narcissist has to very quickly stamp out the scapegoat personality or lose control of the family. They do this by blaming and criticising the scapegoat for everything. When I say everything, I mean everything. You get the blame for being born. You will get the blame for everything that goes wrong in the narcissist's life. You are the proverbial cat that gets kicked, the doormat that the narcissist wipes their shoes on and the toilet that the narcissist uses without flushing. You are criticised for everything you do. If you ever step out of your role as scapegoat and attempt to do something for yourself you are ridiculed into submission. Know your place. In this environment the scapegoat has no means in which to develop a healthy self-esteem. Based on the evidence it is easy for the scapegoat to conclude that if their own parents tell them on a daily basis that they are 'shit' then that must be the case. Scapegoat children have huge issues with their self-esteem, imposter syndrome and feeling unworthy of love and affection.

The Missing Child is just that: missing. One day they pack what little they have and disappear. The missing child would rather take their chances on the streets if need be than suffer at the hands of their narcissist parents. Sometimes they travel to the furthest place on the planet, somewhere where they cannot to be found. You may see the missing child in old photos but you will never see them in real life. The missing child often has issues around fitting in and connecting with others. They are often loners.

The Sacrificial Lamb is the child that sacrifices themselves for the narcissist parent. We are all familiar with the concept of sacrifice. Many of us sacrifice a holiday because we want to buy a car. Or we may sacrifice going out because we have bills to pay. But imagine if someone else tells you what you should sacrifice. That is a bitter pill to take. The narcissist parent tells the child that they will be a doctor, a lawyer or an accountant just because the narcissist wants bragging rights. The child might have to go into the family business just because the narcissist says so and they will not hear otherwise. The child must sacrifice their passion for the narcissist. The sacrificial lamb might have to sacrifice love. They meet someone and fall in love but the narcissist parent is having none of it. They tell the sacrificial lamb to break up with the love of their life or they will be cut off, disinherited and ostracised from the entire family. I am sure Hollywood is full of children that sacrificed their childhoods because their narcissistic parent wanted to be rich and famous and they are doing it vicariously through their child. It happens way too often that when these child stars become adults and their careers dry up; they suffer with massive identity crisis.

The Slave Child is the one that washes, cooks, clean and irons for the family. They look after siblings, babysit and fetch and carry. The slave ends up being the martyr doing everything for everybody else. You will always find the slave child in the kitchen at parties. The slave child is a martyr and a people pleaser. If the slave child doesn't escape they will end up being the caregiver for their narcissist parent in old age.

The Golden Child. The narcissist chooses the golden child because they see something in the golden child that they approve of. It could be that the child looks like them. Maybe they are attractive or have a skill or talent. The golden child is responsible for the success of the family whether they like it or not. It may seem like they got off lightly but many golden children do not.

They get bullied and pushed into achieving the goals of the narcissist so that they can bask in their reflected glory. The golden child realises that in order to stay on the good side of the narcissist parent they had better do their bidding. They can see that their siblings are treated like shit and so they fight really hard to stay top dog. They terrorise their siblings on the narcissist's behalf, they snitch on them and throw them under the bus when necessary. The golden child is always performing and being obsequious. In reality they have no idea who they are and their performance is a mask which hides the emptiness they feel inside.

The Lost Child is the child that gets completely ignored. The narcissist doesn't have much of an imagination. They allocate roles and assignments to their children but if another child comes along and they run out of roles they will simply ignore the child. You have heard the phase 'children should be seen and not heard'; in the case of the lost child, the child is seen and then every effort is made to show the child that they are not seen. The narcissist parent never speaks to the lost child directly. So they might say in front of the lost child to the golden child 'Tell your brother that their dinner is on the table'. The lost child is withdrawn and socially awkward.

The Comedy Child is not allocated this role by the narcissist. The narcissist doesn't understand comedy. The comedy child takes it upon themselves to be the entertainment and comic relief for the toxic family. The comedy child is smart and they realise very early on that they can distract the narcissist by doing something stupid, making a fool of themselves or attempting to make the narcissist laugh. The narcissist has a very childish sense of humour. So they enjoy cartoons. The comedy child is always laughing and cracking jokes but the painted on smile is a cover for the burden of having to make everyone happy all the time. The comedy child makes everyone laugh and inside they are dying. I think of all the children of narcissists it is the comedy child who is more likely to do harm to themselves. Behind the painted smile is a world of depression.

None of the roles I have described are permanent. There is no sentimentality when it comes to the narcissist reallocating roles for their children. If one of their offspring leaves, then the narcissist reallocates that role to another child.

If you are the only child then you will have to double or triple up on roles. If you are the golden child you will easily fall from grace if you get physically injured, crack under the pressure of being perfect all the time or you become ill.

The narcissist cannot abide sickness. Other people's sickness really irritates them. Firstly because it takes all the attention off them and secondly they know how they play the victim when they are sick and they don't believe that anyone could be genuinely ill. The scapegoat, because of their personality, tends to always be the scapegoat but they might become the slave if something happens to the slave. The sacrificial lamb could become the golden child if they forget their own dreams and succeed in whatever profession the narcissist wants them to succeed in. The lost child is a contender to be the scapegoat or the slave if need be. The missing child could become the golden child if they return home and have done something that the narcissist approves of.

Your parents had one job and that was to show you the way to being a well-adjusted emotionally intelligent human being and they messed it up. That isn't your fault. How is that your fault? Don't take it personally. It had nothing to do with you. A narcissist is a narcissist first and foremost; it has nothing to do with you. Your parent is a narcissist over being your parent. A narcissist is who they are and a parent is a role they are given. Just because they are a parent and they are required to feed you and clothe you doesn't mean that they will ever be a loving mother or father to you.

Child abuse is a crime against humanity. Child abuse is messy. Child abuse is confusing. Child abuse is evil. Child abuse changes your brain chemistry. Growing up in a toxic environment means that a child is always in a state of fight, flight, freeze and appease. This makes the child hypervigilant and supersensitive. The travesty of child abuse is that the child is robbed. They are robbed of knowing who they are and who they might have become. The word 'parent' according to Latin means 'to bring forth'. Your parents bring you into this world and the unspoken rule is that they will set you on the right path to be a well-adjusted human being. The narcissist parent barely makes it as a human themselves and so the child stands little chance of learning the skills required to be human. The children of narcissists, regardless of the roles they were assigned to take, are destined to live a life of struggle within themselves and with the world around them.

There are no words to describe child abuse. Child abuse is an oxymoron. To put those two words together is a contradiction in terms. The words are inadequate to describe the suffering. The words take on a different meaning when your parent is your abuser. The very idea that the person who brought you in the world is indifferent to your existence and has no interest in your development is a mind fuck of the highest order. It is a mind fuck and a shit show from start to finish.

In a healthy nurturing environment a child is encouraged to be who they are. This gives the child a sense of identity. When a child is shown love they develop self-worth. If they are encouraged to find out what they are good at and go for their dreams, no matter how crazy, they will develop courage and self-esteem. If they are taught strong values then they will come to know what is right for them, what is wrong for them and learn about boundaries and self-respect. In a healthy environment the child develops emotional intelligence. They are encouraged to express their emotions freely.

The abused child stands no chance of expressing their emotions. I often ask my clients about their emotions and feelings. They tell me they feel numb. This is because their emotions are blocked, entangled and fused together. Numbness is not a feeling. Numbness is an ego defence mechanism. Numbness protects you from pain and damage. Numbness occurs when the system shuts down. Numbness is what you get when the system goes into shock. It is an ego defence mechanism against pain. I want you to know that numbness is not the final destination. Numbness exists to protect you.

On Monday we spoke about the narcissist personality disorder. The narcissist that you are dealing with is disordered. It isn't a matter of whether they are disordered or not, it is more a matter of to what extent are they disordered. If you want to waste your life trying to fix them or appease them and that's up to you but you need to know that you are dealing with someone with a recognised clinical disorder. Anything you do will not work in the way you want it to work.

I want to stop here for the evening but before I do what questions do you have?"

"I have a question. You said earlier on that the narcissist develops narcissism as a defensive mechanism against child abuse. But many of us here suffered child abuse and we didn't become narcissists. Could you say some more about this?"

"Sure! All of us are different. No two of us are the same. We may have suffered similar abuse but the impact will be different. Some people were abused as children and merrily declare that it didn't do them any harm. Others are abused and they never get over it. They take the abuse with them to the grave. It isn't what happens to you in life that is the deciding factor on how your life will turn out. It is what you make of what happened to you that determines how your life will turn out. Some people become people pleasers. Others become recluses. The narcissist decides to become a narcissist.

I am reminded of the Navy Seal David Goggins whose father beat him every day and on a couple of occasions put young David in hospital. Growing up David witnessed his father beat his mother up and when he had done beating up his mother he would turn on him. Today, David Goggins is recognised as the toughest man alive. Among other exploits he runs 150 miles a week. Goggins is also a formidable motivational speaker and he says that he had to grow 'callouses on his mind' otherwise his father would have killed him.

The bottom line is that if you are dealing with a narcissist you are dealing with damaged goods. The narcissist is a bruised child who made a pact with an imaginary friend called the devil. In return for perfection they would provide the devil with supply. The devil being the devil tricked the narcissist. The devil failed to tell the narcissist that as part of the deal they would never be free of the feelings of self-loathing and that they were fated to walk this earth doing the devil's work and endlessly feeding them with supply from unsuspecting souls".

"Did I ever love the narcissist? I am so confused".

"That's a good question but how do I know whether you loved the narcissist or not. I am not you. Well actually I do know but let me ask you a few questions so that you get to know too.

"What is love?"

"I don't know"

"So how can you ask me whether you loved the narcissist or not when you don't even know what love is in the first place. Maybe you were in love with the idea of love? Ok let me ask you this.

Do you love yourself?"

"No"

"Then how can you love anyone if you do not love yourself? You cannot give what you do not have to give". OK.

Were you abused as a child?"

"Yes"

"Maybe your idea of love is drama, trauma and abuse. I would say that it isn't love that you feel for the narcissist. It is familiarity.

Consider this: what you feel towards the narcissist is limerence. You didn't fall in love, you fell in limerence.

According to psychologist Dorothy Tennov, limerence is a phenomenon that mimics love. If you are in limerence with someone you become obsessed with the person. You think that you cannot live without this person. You need them in order to breathe.

I am going to give you six features of limerence relationships and then we will go back to your original question.

-YOU THINK THAT THE NARCISSIST IS THE MISSING LINK TO YOUR LIFE. THEY COMPLETE YOU JUST LIKE THEY SAY IN THE MOVIES.

-YOU WANT THEM WHETHER THEY ARE GOOD FOR YOU OR NOT AND NO MATTER HOW THEY TREAT YOU.

-YOU CONTINUE TO IGNORE THE RED FLAGS.

-YOU NEGLECT OYUR NEEDS FOR THEM.

-YOU CANNOT FUNCTION IF OYU DO NOT KNOW WHERE THEY ARE AND WHAT THEY WHAT THEY'RE DOING.

-ALL SAID AND DONE YOU REALLY DON'T' KNOW THAT MUCH ABOUT THEM.

"So now I am going to ask you the original question you asked me.

Did you ever love the narcissist? And your answer is?"

"*No*".

"Case closed".

"*All of us here have been through some sort of abuse and are probably suffering from PTSD. What are your views on PTSD and what can we do about it*"?

Let me answer you by telling you about this man I meet from time to time when walking my dog. I'll call him Sam. You know how it is, at first you say "hello" and then the hello moves to "How are you" and then before long you are actually having a full blown conversation. Sam was in the army and suffers from PTSD. He told me that he has to walk for miles every day to even out his mind. He was institutionalised for two years. They put him on medication which turned him into a zombie. PTSD ruined his life. Unfortunately for Sam, doctors didn't recognise PTSD before 1980. Before that time PTSD was called 'shell shock'. Sufferers were told to 'get over it' and 'pull themselves together'.

The medical profession says that there is no cure for PTSD. I beg to differ. How you deal with PTSD in my opinion is not by giving pills and potions that suppress the disorder. I think the way to deal with PTSD is to deal with it. Head on. As terrifying as it may be, it isn't going away until you face it.

PTSD or post-traumatic stress disorder can occur when a person has been exposed to something so traumatic that the brain blows a fuse. When you suffer with anxiety it is because you have a fear of something happening that hasn't happened yet. With PTSD something has happened. The brain has the evidence.

Any horrific experience can give a person PTSD. It can be rape, violence, witnessing or being in a car accident, being mugged or having your home burgled. PTSD can develop from any situation where the person feels that their life is at risk.

The symptoms of PTSD sit on top of anxiety and depression. That is to say if you already suffer with anxiety and depression, PTSD will give you another set of symptoms to deal with. The symptoms include nightmares, night terrors and hallucinations. But the distinguishing feature of PTSD is the flashbacks. The sufferer's brain takes them right back into the traumatic event and they may relive that trauma spontaneously at any time or place. It is terrifying. The thing with PSTD is that anything could trigger you. The onset of PTSD is usually about six weeks after the exposure to trauma. Having said that it can show up at any time. PTSD can last up to two years or a lifetime.

The trauma you went through is in every muscle of your body. Call it muscle memory. Anything can trigger your body to react. I have been banging on about having treatments this week. A powerful way of getting trauma out of your cells, out of your muscles and bones and finally out of your head is to do body work. It sounds counterintuitive but it works. Body work is the fastest, safest and cheapest way to reset your brain. Any kind of body work that gets you moving is going to repair your body. Dance, sport, exercise, spa, massage, gym. It doesn't matter what you do as long as you do something.

All of you have been having treatments here at the resort and I guarantee that you are sleeping better and waking up refreshed. Every day that you are here you are getting stronger.

Now that you know pretty much all that you need to know about the narcissist, you have some decisions to make about the narcissist you are dealing with.

I hope you decide that you are not going to let anyone tell you who you are or how to live your life. Especially if that person is disordered. What do they know? I hope you decide that you are not going to allow others to roam around in your head, rent free, controlling everything you do and don't do. I hope you decide that the suffering is over. I hope you choose you. Tonight as you relax play with these questions.

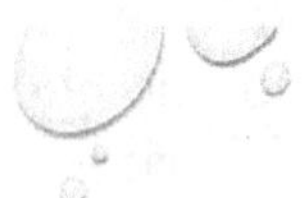

Let's finish here for today.

As you know, tomorrow the workshop is outside. The resort has set up the workshop at my favourite part of the beach. I call it 'the cove'.

Can we meet at 8.30 am tomorrow at reception? Good! We will be conducting a 'silent walk' on our way to the cove. Silent walks are amazing for clearing the chattering mind. When we meet up tomorrow please greet each other with a smile, a nod or a hug but no talking. Not one word should pass your lips until we reach our destination. OK? Good.

You do not need to bring anything. All provisions will be there. They say it will rain tomorrow. I hope it does.

See you tomorrow..."

WEDNESDAY

THE BEACH

Bev was in reception just before 8.30.

As people approached she put her finger to her lips. 'Shhhhh' Silence. They took the trail out of the resort that led to the beach. The morning was fresh. The sun was not quite there but they could feel it coming. It was going to be a hot one. For some reason they walked in single file. Together and alone. Connected but detached.

After about 45 minutes of walking they arrived at the cove. A rock jutting out the cliff provided the roof and shelter. An old disused boat housed a coolbox that contained all the goodies that they needed for the day. Think of how you imagine a beautiful beach setting to be and the cove was it. They each chose a sun lounger and flopped down on it.

After a long while Bev spoke.

"Healing is here today...so let's heal.

I have brought you here so that you can make some important decisions about your life and who you want to have in it. You can leave all your fears here on this beach or carry them around with you forever more. The decision is yours. We will carry out a number of rituals that can free you from your entanglement with the narcissist. When you walk back from here you will be walking the long road to freedom. You have earned your freedom. You deserve freedom.

I was taught many lessons from an amazing woman called Denise Linn. Look her up on Google when you get home. I attended many of her classes before she became a famous international speaker. She is Native American from the Cherokee tribe. She taught me how to conduct past live regression, cellular rejuvenation and many more healing methods that were handed down to her from the elders of her tribe. The silent walk we just did is one of her teachings. When you walk in silence with no distractions or input from anyone else you are alone with your thoughts. The miracle of the silent walk is that once you are alone with your thoughts you realise that under the chaos of your thoughts is peace and stillness. Do you agree? They all nodded. They were completely chilled out.

Peace is in your nature. Underneath chaos is peace.

You will heal by telling your version of your story today. Storytelling is an ancient human art form.

You tell the story. You hear the story. You tell the story and you correct the story. When you tell the story you find out that the story doesn't impress you anymore. You tell your story and it loses its grip on you. The story doesn't define who you are. You tell a different story. There is also magic in telling your story to others who can listen without prejudice.

You tell your story, you expose the wound and the energies of the group heal you. They heal you because no matter how terrifying your story is, they heal you with kindness, understanding, validation and acceptance.

We are going to use the 'talking stick'. Bev held up the talking stick for them all to see.

The carvings on the stick tell a story of truth and it compels you to speak your truth. When someone is in possession of the talking stick, listen. When you listen, listen with your heart and you will find something magical happen. It is called healing. When one person tells their story and shares their pain, you will notice that their story is actually your story. You will hear the same story of abuse over and over again today. As you listen you will notice that your story loses its power over you.

Tell your story here today and leave it here today."

Bev gave the talking stick to Harshida.

Harshida was hesitant.

"It sucks to go first...

They were all silent. Slowly she found her voice and began to speak.

"He said he loved my hair. In the beginning he would spend hours stroking my hair. What man does that? I thought he was my dream come true. You know just like the movies. After the wedding, it went downhill fast. It wasn't a gradual change, it was almost overnight. He didn't have to pretend anymore. He was Mr Nice Guy to everyone except me. He had a kind word for everybody except me. Raj was the guy that would do anything for anyone. You needed money, ask Raj. You needed advice, ask Raj. You needed a place to stay, ask Raj. Everyone in the community loved him.

Most nights Raj raped me. He had condoms in his bedside cabinet, openly on show for me to see but he never had time to put a condom on when he raped me. The condoms were for his extramarital activities.

Tears streamed down Harshida's face.

He would sit downstairs like a fat deranged Buddha watching porn and breathing heavily. The image of him sitting there makes my skin crawl.

"Come and sit beside me" he would say, "You might learn a few tricks". He mocked me. He laughed in contempt and glee at the same time.

After he had overdosed on porn and whiskey he'd come upstairs and degrade me. One time he watched a movie, heaven knows where he got it from. It was about men pissing on women for kicks. It think it is called the golden shower. He did that to me.”

Harshida's body was shaking. She couldn't get her words out so she howled instead. Her face contorted in pain but she kept going...

"He came into the bedroom, held me down and pissed on me. The hair that he said he loved so much... he pissed on it.

Do you know what he said to me after? "He said "You're worthless. You aren't worth my piss. Clean yourself up... you're a 'pisshead'. The fucker laughed at his own joke for the rest of the night.

What is the matter with me? I used to be so brave. I have a master's degree in fine arts. I am a teacher for fuck's sake. At first he told me he was proud of me because I was so smart. Then he made fun of my qualifications saying that no one wanted a useless artist like me. I proved him wrong. Someone did employ me and I was doing very well. That was the first time I saw his temper. I came home and cooked dinner and told him that I had been promoted. I expected him to be happy for me, for us. Instead he went into a rage. He told me that he wanted a wife to look after him and the house. If I was in this new job I would be working all hours of the day and night and I wouldn't be able to keep house. It never occurred to him that he could do something around the house. I tried to reassure him that I could do both.

That night he raped me. He raped me every night for a week. I fell pregnant and had to turn down the promotion.

After our son was born he left me alone. No more rape. No more anything. He barely talked to me let alone touch me. He still sat on the sofa watching porn, drinking whiskey. The condoms were regularly topped up so I knew that he was getting sex elsewhere. I was relieved.

My relief didn't last long. He started beating me. Every time he came anywhere near me, I flinched. I am a nervous wreck. My body aches all over. I can't sleep. I can't eat. I can't concentrate. I can't remember anything. I am not interested in anything. I have no motivation to do anything. I am the living dead.

If you saw this fucker out in public you would swear he was the most amazing man you've ever met. He's the life and soul of any party. He buys everyone drinks when we are out. He loves to play it large. People think that we have a lovely lifestyle. We don't. We are up to our eyeballs in debt and he doesn't give a shit about anything other than his dick.

I tried to talk to my own mother and she basically told me to shut up and stop making a fuss. I don't know what possessed me to talk to her. She is fairly and squarely on his side. She is in his pocket. In fact every member of my family and friends is in his pocket. My own mother betrayed me. He sent flying monkeys to spy on me. I became paranoid. He made it so that I was the crazy one and he was the long-suffering husband, admired by all for putting up with my mad behaviour.

Do you know, I tried to leave him once? I thought to myself that since he didn't even notice me that he wouldn't notice if I left. I had no clue where I was going to go and I didn't have a lot of money. I was desperate. Well, he came home early from work on the flipping day that I had decided to leave.

He saw all the bags and immediately put two and two together. He leapt at me. He was at the front door and I was at the end of the hallway and in one move he punched me. The punch landed across my jaw and shoulder. The whole side of my body went numb. He then grabbed me by my hair and pulled me up the stairs to the spare bedroom. I still have the carpet burns on my back to this day. He opened the door and threw me in. I stayed in the spare room for seventeen days and seventeen nights.

During those seventeen days he gave me water and a little food. He allowed me to go to the bathroom once a day. Sometimes it was mornings, sometimes it was late in the night. I asked him if I could have a chamber pot and then he wouldn't have to worry about taking me to the bathroom. This idea seemed to please him and so the next day he threw a bucket into the room. It seemed like a good idea at the time but that bucket became my nemesis. After about three days that bucket stank so bad that it made me wretch to go near it.

My God was I at rock bottom. For seventeen days I didn't brush my teeth. I couldn't take a shower and I didn't change my clothes. Every day was endless. I regressed. I cried. I ruminated, I saw patterns on the wall and I talked to the patterns on the wall. I heard voices outside as people passed by. When I heard voices I kept quiet. I was still more concerned with keeping up appearances. I was more concerned with what others thought of me.

How could I be so concerned about what other people thought of me when I thought nothing of myself? After the seventeen days he let me go. He only let me go because our son was coming home from university. He knew I was broken. He told me with dead eyes if I ever tried to leave him again then he would track me down and kill me. The police would find my charred body in a suitcase in a ditch somewhere. This freaked me out because this is exactly what happened to an Indian woman called Kiran Daudia.

After a beating he liked to hold me down. He literally sat on my body so I couldn't move and he would tell me in graphic detail how he would chop my body up piece by piece if I ever pulled a stunt like trying to leave again. After one of his stories I couldn't sleep. All thoughts of leaving him left me.

I often thought about killing myself. I didn't even care what my suicide would do to my son. I was too far gone to care. The only reason why I didn't carry it out was because I knew that he would dine out on my death. The community would rally around him and it wouldn't be too long before he claimed another slave. I replaced the idea of killing myself with the idea of killing him. I ruminated over it. I relished every little detail in my head.

God forgive me for thinking such dreadful thoughts. This was how I would do it. I would wait until he was slightly inebriated and well into his porn. I would walk up to him casually and plunge a bread knife into his belly and twist it so he couldn't get it out. I would sit down with a cup of tea and watch him bleed to death. I would sit there and watch the terror in his eyes. I would listen to his cries for help. Those were the thoughts that comforted me to sleep most nights.

I am afraid for my safety but more than that I am afraid of what he is turning me into. I am a monster with murder on her mind. I am afraid that one day I will walk into the kitchen, get the bread knife, walk into the lounge and plunge the knife into his big fat belly. Every time I get a beating, I'd take myself off to fantasy land where I am stabbing him over and over again with a bread knife.

You cannot believe the lies I had to tell to be here this week. As far as he is concerned I am in hospital right now sorting out a female issue. Oh God...what has my life become..."

The group was openly crying now. Harshida's dam had burst. All the years of having to be strong and playing happy family had collapsed. VJ took her hand. For a moment he wished he hadn't made that move, because Harshida was squeezing the circulation out of his fingers. Harshida squeezed and VJ held on.

"Take deep breaths Harshida.... Listen to me. Breathe. Everyone follow me. Breathe in for five. Hold it for five. Breathe out slowly for five. Where there is breath, there is life and where there is life there is hope.

Let it all go Harshida. We are all here. We hear you. We see you. We feel your pain. Your pain is our pain. You have done a wonderful thing. By speaking out you have given everyone here permission to speak out too. You have given everyone here a gift. Thank you".

Everyone found that they were following Bev's words. They breathed in and breathed out. It occurred to more than one of them that their breath was like the ebb and flow of the tide. They didn't know it at the time but they were tuning in to the healing powers of nature.

Without knowing why, VJ took the talking stick from Harshida. He never let go of her hand.

After a long while. VJ spoke.

"For the first time in my life I feel calm. For years I thought it was me that was strange. Why did I not fit in? Why did I always feel strange around my family? To be honest, I have never shared this with anyone, my family gave me the creeps. When you spoke about the Cluster B family on Monday, you were essentially talking about my family. Cluster B meet the Kumars.

My father, he that must be obeyed, is the psychopath. My mother is a narcissist and my brother and sister are both sociopaths. My family makes a lot of money from selling land in India that doesn't exist. People lose their life savings and my father gets away with it all the time. By the time these people have invested their money they have nothing left to pay a lawyer. My father always laughs it off by saying that people should always read the small print.

His thing is money. He is absolutely obsessed with making money. From the moment I was born my parents took one look at me and decided that they didn't like me. I couldn't figure out why. Everything my sister did was OK with them. Anything from torturing next door's cat to setting fire to the sofa. One day she found some money on the table, she took it and then proceeded to burn the notes on the stove. The look on her face as she saw the money go up in flames was pure evil. She was in ecstasy. She told me to try it and like a trusting fool I did. At that precise moment my father walked in to the room. Needless to say he beat the shit out of me. He beat me with *his belt and the buckle gashed my arm. I got ten stitches that day. They didn't even want to take me to the hospital. It was only after they became concerned that I was going to bleed out that they reluctantly took me. The story they told the doctors was that I had banged into a door. The doctors looked at me and I looked at them. We both knew it was bullshit.*

My brother is a piece of work. He drives around in fancy cars and wears snazzy suits. All of which are bought from scamming innocent people out of their hard earned money. He gets on the phone and talks vulnerable people into hare-brained deals. He has literally made millions. During the pandemic he made an absolute fortune by setting up a bogus company that could transport masks and PPE gear from China to the west. He sold millions of masks that never arrived.

My brother and his wife live in the same house as my parents. My parents thought it was a good idea to marry him off so that they could have a lavish wedding and show everyone how prosperous they were. They all went off to India to make a marriage deal. They found an 18 year old girl from a village. Plucked her from her family and married her into slavery and debauchery. The wedding had a thousand guests. It was held over four days and over three continents. Can you imagine how many people got scammed to pay for my brother's wedding? My sister- in-law never talks but at night I hear her crying out. My brother is a monster.

For a long time I thought I was the scapegoat, but somehow the label didn't fit. Yes, I got the blamed for everything. Whether I was there or not didn't seem to matter. When you spoke about the sacrificial lamb in yesterday's class, everything fell into place. I am the sacrificial lamb.

You know what my dearest mummy did? Of course you don't. She dressed me up in girl's clothes. Despite my obvious anatomy she dressed me up as a girl. She wanted a girl. I became the girl.

When people asked her about me, she told them that it was me that wanted to dress up as a girl and she was allowing me to express myself.

People looked upon her as the perfect mother. In the community she was caring and tolerant. At home she would threaten me into submission until I put on a flipping dress. I started wearing girls' clothes for an easier life. Most people I'd meet thought I was a girl until the beard starting showing".

He laughed. They laughed.

"When I was fourteen, my mother announced that I was gay. Just like that. I wouldn't have a problem with being gay if I was gay, but I'm not. My mother decided my gender and then my sexuality. Is that a decision for someone else to make?

I was called every name you could imagine at school, in the streets and at home. There was no peace. I used to sit alone in my room in the darkness and pray to die. Sometimes I'd sneak a knife from the kitchen and in my room I'd play with it as if it was a toy.

It started off as play and then accidentally but on purpose I started to draw blood.

I used to cut myself and watch the blood trickle down my arm. It was the weirdest thing but it was better to feel the pain that the knife inflicted than to feel the pain in my heart. For me cutting was a distraction and it was release. I felt in control and a sense of power. I had a secret that they knew nothing about and it made me feel good. I used physical pain to relieve emotional pain. It worked for a while but cutting myself wasn't enough. I wanted to die. I recognise that self-harming was one step removed from killing myself. I was practising for the main event".

VJ fell silent. He was motionless apart from a single vein that pulsed angrily in his temple.

Harshida whispered the Gayathri Mantra under her breath. Everyone heard it but only VJ understood it. He closed his eyes and melted into her voice.

Sarah took the talking stick.

"Do you know the worst thing my mother ever said to me? Well of course you don't. Nobody does.

I was sitting on the bed watching her get ready to go somewhere.

As usual she was in a mood. She suddenly turned to me.

'Sarah... you are years of nothing.'

I had no clue what she meant by that. I looked at her. She became even more frustrated as she realised that her words had no effect on me. So she went in for the kill.

'I wish you had never been born'. Her words had reached their target. She smiled.

From that day on everything made sense. She didn't want me let alone love me. I stood no chance.

My so-called mother hounded me. She criticised, judged and ridiculed my every move. I was a child under siege. She berated me. She hated me. According to her I was the reason why she hadn't seen the world. I was the reason why she had to wear cheap clothes. She'd say 'I have to wear this old coat because I have to buy you clothes and shoes'.

The irony was that she had the latest fashion. Her nails and hair were always immaculate, but if I needed something new for school or because I had happened to grow out of it, she would go ballistic.

My mother always wore inappropriate clothes. Low cut dresses, tight jumpers. She had her *boobs done when I was nine and that meant that we didn't eat a decent meal until the loan on the boobs had been paid for. She used to swan around the town in the most ridiculous clothes with me in tow. She acted as if I didn't belong to her. When people were around she would refer to herself in the third person.*

'Now come along Sarah or your mother will get upset.' Who talks like that other than a crazy person?

I took a beating for everyone that had done her wrong in her life. When she was beating me with whatever she could find it was as if she was having an out of body experience. Her eyes would turn black and her face would contort. I swear she looked possessed. With every slap, punch or kick she'd bring up people that had done this and that to her. She remembered everyone in detail and so the beatings were long and drawn out. She would start ranting about someone or other and her own temper would lose its temper.

I was the reason why she hadn't pursued her career. I was the reason why she was stuck with my 'good for nothing fucking father.'

She never referred to my father as 'your father'. My father was known as 'your fucking father'. His full title was 'your fucking good for nothing lowdown piece of shit father'.

One time when I was at kindergarten, they asked us to draw a picture of our family. The teacher came around and asked each of us to describe who was in the picture. When it was my turn I stood up and showed my picture to the rest of the class. I said innocently 'this is my mother and this is my 'fucking father'. I didn't know that that wasn't his name. The teacher went into shock. I repeated myself and explained that that the person in the drawing was my 'fucking good for nothing piece of shit father'. When she came to she marched me to the principal's office. My mother was hauled in. She was sweetness and light. 'Oh I don't know where she got that sort of language from'. She apologised to the teacher and reassured them that it would never happen again. All the way home she called me every name under the sun. She then told me that I was just like my "fucking father".

Sarah laughed.

"What a fucking joke".

She laughed some more. Everyone laughed. Suddenly she started to cry. Everyone started to cry. She laughed and she was off again.

"She would blow hot and cold. I never knew in advance how my mother would react to a situation. If I did something that she didn't like I would get the beating of my life. She loved to tell me in advance how she was going to beat me.

"I am going to beat your backside 'til it bleeds'. 'Just wait until we get home".

Often when we got home she would watch a bit of telly or go on social media. I would hope and pray that she had forgotten or forgiven me. That never happened. Even when we had visitors she would act like the perfect mother. I was expected to smile and get the biscuits like a dutiful daughter. After the visitors left, she would beat the shit out of me. My mother would burst into my bedroom. Her style would be to fling open the door so violently it would bang against the wall. This she knew would frighten the shit out of me. She stood in the door winding herself up by relaying exactly what I had done and how disrespectful I had been to her. Then she would beat me with whatever she had in her hand. A belt. A stick. It wasn't so much the beating that terrified me. It was the waiting for the beating that was the worst. She knew that and she loved it.

My mother told me repeatedly that I would never amount to anything. She used to tell me on a regular basis how I had ruined her life. I was the reason she didn't go to university. I was the reason why she didn't travel the world. I get the blame for things that happened to her before I was born.

At every opportunity she would dump me with my grandparents. Staying at my grandparents was torture. I used to look out the window willing my mother to come and get me. One day, and I remember it as if it was yesterday, I was looking out the window. Underneath the window was an old rusty radiator that didn't work properly. Nothing in my grandparents' house worked. On this particular day I climbed up on it to see out. After a while my legs started to cramp, but because I had lost all sensation in my legs, I miscalculated getting down. My leg caught on the jagged edge of the radiator and sliced open. Blood spewed out of my leg and at the same time my mother arrived.

She looked at me with rage and cursed me. She took me home, slapped my face and sent me to bed. In the morning we had to go to the hospital because someone told her that I should have a tetanus injection just in case. She scolded me all the way to the hospital, in the waiting room and all the way home again. When I think of it, I got abused simply because I was wanting my mother but she didn't want me. I was a total inconvenience to her.

My mother never had a good word to say about me or to me unless we were in public. When we met any of the neighbours she would go on about my grades at school. But as soon as we got in the house she would call the neighbours 'nosy fuckers'. She conveniently forgot that she was the one who bragged about everything. I was the scapegoat, the sacrificial lamb and the golden child all in one.

She fucked up my life entirely. You know what the saddest thing is? I have a PHD for goodness sake but I have no idea who I am. She hated the fact that I was smart. She resented the fact that I had an opportunity to study. She loved to show off about the fact that I had got into a good university. I remember on the way to the awards ceremony she called me a 'stupid bitch' because I had taken the wrong turning off the motorway. Throughout the ceremony people came up to congratulate us and she lapped it up. She even used the royal 'we'. She and I had just completed a PHD. On the way home she called me 'stupid bitch' again for something that I had or hadn't done.

I realise now that I could never please her because she didn't see me as a person in my own right. I was an extension of her. When she spoke to me she was actually speaking to herself. The venom with which she lashed out to me on a daily basis was her way of letting blood and feeling better about herself."

Geordie took the talking stick.

"My mother lives in sheltered accommodation. I don't see her. Yet even though I haven't seen her for years I am eaten up with guilt for not seeing her. She still lives in my head. I have no self-esteem because of her. I have no friends because of her. I can't trust anyone. I am too scared to try anything because of her. She ruined my life.

A while ago I tried to have a conversation with her. I wanted her to know what she had done to me. I don't know what I was expecting. An apology perhaps. She went ballistic. She started screaming that I was trying to kill her. All the care home assistants came running. Once again she brought shame on me. A nurse told me to leave and I haven't been back.

I am tormented by what she did to me. How can a mother not love her own child? All around me I see mothers loving their children. Why couldn't she love me? What did I do that was so wrong that turned my own mother against me?

I tried everything to get her attention. She knew it. In fact she revelled in it. The more I tried to get her attention the more she would give it to others. She loved other people's children and hated her own daughter.

Do you know that every night I'd pray for my real mother to appear? Surely the ranting harpy that I lived with couldn't possibly be my mother. I convinced myself that there must have been a mix up at the hospital and I landed with the family from hell.

There are chunks of my childhood that I do not remember at all. The brain saves you from the detail, I guess. You get snippets and flashbacks that you can't piece together. I was there but I wasn't there. My childhood was an out of body experience. I nearly said experiment. There's a Freudian slip for you. I think when a child is abused the spirit takes the child somewhere else. It's a form of child protection.

My mother is mad. I see that now. You say disordered, I call it madness. It wasn't her fault but I was the one who paid for it. She was the product of an abusive family. My grandparents on her side were something else. Every summer I stayed with them in their tiny cottage that stank of piss. It was awful. By day I had to listen to my grandmother spit venom about everyone and by night I had to lie there and pretend to be asleep while my grandfather molested me. My grandfather would come in the room. I still shudder at the thought of his arthritic bony fingers all over me".

She shuddered as if to prove the point. They all shuddered in unison.

"He had little movement in his hands. It felt like he was mauling me. His fingers were claws. One night I don't know what made me do it but I decided to open my eyes. Maybe I thought that if my grandfather saw that I was awake he would come to his senses and stop. I opened my eyes and looked into the abyss. His eyes were two black holes. He was the devil. From then on I kept my eyes tightly shut. I played dead. His breath was disgusting.

If you are there only to abuse your own granddaughter at least brush your teeth, you pig. His breath smelt of rotting flesh and whiskey. To this day I go into a cold sweat if I smell whisky.

At night I would spend hours trying to figure out where to place my head so that I didn't have to breathe in his air. I didn't realise until now that I was more concerned about getting away from his rancid breath than the fact that he molested me.

My mother treated him with complete contempt. I don't know if he had molested her as well when she was young, but by the way she spoke to him and the way she treated me, I am pretty sure that he did.

When he died no one went to his funeral. My mother didn't go because she had a Zumba class that day and she didn't want to miss it. My grandmother couldn't go because she had lost her mind to dementia. If anyone had turned up to his funeral it wouldn't be because they wanted to pay their last respects, it would be to make sure he was dead".

Break

"We have heard your stories so far. I am so sorry for your pain. No child deserves to go through what you went through. The words 'child abuse' seem inadequate to describe what you all have suffered. It is almost too much to comprehend that the person who gave life to you is also your abuser. But know this: whoever abused you did it because they are troubled and damaged souls. If they knew any better they would do better. They abused you because they are in pain and the only way to discharge the pain is to make someone feel worse.

It is the way of the child to take it personally and think 'I am the reason why my parents are so angry and hateful towards me'. It is the way of the child to think that there is something wrong with them and that is why their parents can't show them love. It is the way of the child to think that they are not worthy of love.

It is the way of the abused child to carry the feelings of inadequacy into adulthood. The abuse they received at the hands of their parents or siblings defines their every move.

How on earth are you responsible for the behaviour of a narcissist that happens to be your parent? I want you to make a decision about this today. This shit stops here. Enough is enough. As a child you did nothing wrong. I don't think it helps you to think of your mother as a narcissist. I think you should think of your mother as a narcissist who happens to be your mother. Your mother is a narcissist first and foremost. As brutal as it may seem, loving and supporting you wasn't on her list".

Cynthia kept the stick.

"My family is emotionally constipated. There is nothing there. They are emotional flat-liners. When my uncle died by father put his hand on my shoulder and told me that my uncle was dead and not to cry. The end. I had to piece together the clues in their conversation to find out how he died. I wasn't allowed to go to the funeral. I got it into my head that if Uncle Tommy loved me he

would have taken me with him. I think I stopped trusting people from then on. Everyone that I love always leaves me.

I don't know how it happened but I let him into my life. We both worked together. I am unhappily married and lonely. He was young, free and single. We used to go out for work drinks on a Friday night and I would watch as he worked the room. Cracking a joke here, admiring someone's scarf there. One day it was my turn. He asked if I would like a drink and the rest is history. I had a drink and left the bar with him. We booked into a hotel and stayed there for the whole weekend. That has been my life for the past six years.

I opened myself up to feelings and now I am an addict to those feelings. When he sends me a text, I read it at least ten times. I analyse every word. Just to try and pick up on his mood. I stalk him. He put a device on his phone so that I could see where he is at any given moment. I track him day and night. I torture myself trying to figure out who he's with and whether he will take them home with him. He likes to fuck with me by turning off his phone for an hour or so and then saying,

'You're the one who's married not me'

I have become paranoid. When I go to his place, I am embarrassed to say that I have taken to sniffing the air to see if I can pick up any female smells. Which person in their right mind does the things I do?

Sex with my husband was routine. Saturday night, fumble in the dark, roll over and go to sleep. We had been trying to have children for years but nothing happened. We were on an IVF programme. Sex was a means to an end. The narcissist taught me about sex. In the beginning it was wonderful. Sex was a drug. I couldn't get enough of him.

The irony of what happened next is mind blowing. I fell pregnant with the narcissist's baby at the same time that I was pumping myself with chemicals trying to get pregnant with my husband on an IVF program. The IVF treatment cost twelve grand a shot.

When I told the narcissist that I was pregnant, he said he couldn't be sure the baby was his and so I should get rid of it. So I did. I aborted the baby that I had longed for my whole fucking life. I had to go to a backstreet abortion clinic. If I had gone to the hospital and they had read my notes, I swear they would have sectioned me. I went alone. He didn't come. He said he was too busy.

I have hit rock bottom. I hate myself for letting this happen to me. Do you know what the worst part of it all is? He's not even my type. I used to see him messing around with women in the office and he used to give me the 'ick'.

You know at the Zoom meeting you said that this workshop is not for you if you want tips and tricks on how to get the narcissist to love you. When you said those words you looked directly at me. Even through Zoom you saw through me. I confess that I came on this workshop so that I could learn how to make him love me. I realise now through your teachings that he doesn't even love himself let alone me. He is incapable of love. I cannot save him. I need to save myself. I need to get as far away from him as possible".

The talking stick was passed to James.

"When I married my wife the word narcissist didn't exist. I know it's sexist to say this but I put her mood swings down to her periods. That was the lie I told myself. Because if the lie I told myself were true she would be on her period 365 days of the year. My mother told me not to marry her. It was too late. We had already had sex. For the first year we had sex everywhere and in every position we could think of. She was a free spirit and it made such a difference to my uptight family. Like you, Harshida, as soon as the ring was on her finger I was discarded. My role shifted from partner to banker. She loved to shop and I thought I could make her happy. She wanted breast implants for her birthday. She got them. It became an endless cycle of lip fillers, hair extensions, Botox, nails and whatever was trending on Instagram.

When Covid-19 came along and we couldn't go anywhere or do anything my life took a turn for the worse. All the shops that she loved to visit were closed. She changed literally overnight. It was as if she morphed into another person. She wouldn't let me go near her unless I had done something that she liked. She made me out to be some sort of sex fiend.

The one time that we had sex in 2021 resulted in my son. My life became unbearable. Being cooped up in a small apartment is bad enough but being cooped up with a banshee was too much for me to bear.

She only talked to me if she wanted something. She told me that for one of her birthdays or was it Christmas she wanted a butt lift. This was when I started to wake up. She was considering going to another country to have a serious operation. Who was going to look after our son? When I mentioned this small detail to her, she gave me the silent treatment for weeks. One day I came home from running some errands and she was taking selfies and my son was nowhere to be seen. I finally found him playing with the cat litter tray eating cat shit. That was when I decided enough was enough. I went back home to my family.

I hate myself. I left my defenceless son with a witch. Nobody has to kick me, I kick myself every day. I am a coward, weak and an idiot for marrying her.

After I left her, people started telling me stuff. It turns out that she had sex with half of our wedding party. I was told by a reliable source that she had sex with someone on our wedding night, all I know was that it wasn't with me. Everyone in my town knew about her, but me.

I was the village idiot. I worked all the hours that God sent to give her what she wanted. It was never enough. During lockdown she got the social media bug. She wouldn't get off social media. I swear she was on it eight hours a day. Her phone was surgically attached to her hand. She walked around the house texting, posting and commenting all day long while my son cried in his cot. Many times I came home and had to change the soiled nappy that he had been in all day while she was in the bathroom taking selfies.

I don't care about her anymore but I do care about my son. I am terrified that he is going to end up a narcissist or that she will turn him against me. I now know that the battle between us has nothing to do with my son. It is me she is out to get. She is weaponising my son against me.

For years she made me feel like shit. She has me over a barrel because I am never going to stop caring for my son. I fell into the trap of arguing with her and trying to outwit her. It has been bickering at best and slanging matches at worst. I am ashamed at some of the things I have said in front of my son.

I have realised a few things on this workshop but I need to know if my son is going to be OK."

"James, listen carefully. It is an awful feeling when you have to leave your child in the incapable hands of a narcissist. You had to leave for your own sanity and for your own safety. It is a cliché these days but it is still noteworthy. When you take a flight whom does the flight attendant instruct to buckle up their seatbelt first? You are no use to anyone sick or injured. Your first priority is to your son and that means staying healthy. If something happened to you and you were not able to bring home the bacon then he wouldn't eat. Now that you are out of the toxic environment you can see the situation for what it really is. Do not be afraid that your son will go crazy or turn out to be a narcissist. Your son is your son. He has your blood running through his veins. When he is with you, show him who you are. Teach him how to be a decent human being. She may feed him but she cannot nourish him. You do that. She may give him a bed to sleep in but she cannot give him support and security. You do that. She may criticise and judge him because she cannot love. You show him love. You do all the loving on her behalf. Whatever she does you counter it with love. Never say bad things about her. Do not enter into her world. Your son is growing and what you need to do is provide contrast. You need to show him all that is good so that he can contrast it with evil. He is growing and he will find out who she is without any input from you. Narcissists never win. They die alone. Karma always finds them and dishes them the shit that they dished out for years to others".

James's face crumbled in relief. William took the talking stick from him.

"For most of the week I was wondering if I was in the right workshop. Nothing you said related to

me until you talked about the golden child. I had a lightbulb moment. I had a tyrant for a father, but for some reason that I can never fathom, he favoured me. I was the golden child. I could do no wrong in his eyes. He paraded me around with him as if I was some sort of circus animal.

'Go on Willy boy, show the people your martial arts moves. Go on Willy show them how you can dribble the ball. Willy boy, let's have a song'. I was always a fucking performing seal. All I wanted was for him to leave me alone instead of turning tricks for him.

You might think it's better to be the golden child than a slave or a scapegoat. In a way it's true. I was bullied and there was always a thinly veiled threat that if I didn't perform then I would lose my place. I was never criticised or beaten but my brothers and sisters whom I love were and I had to stand by and watch it. What do you think it did to the relationship I had with my siblings? They hated me. They still do to this day. I don't blame them. They had to listen to my father go on and on about how they should be more like me.

I have come to realise just how much being a golden child has robbed me of me. I don't seem to be able to connect with myself. I am driven. But I don't know what I am driving towards. I achieve goals because that is what I have been programmed to do. I have a high powered job, a lovely house and a fancy car, but it's never enough. I am always shriving for the next big win, thrill, and adventure. I cannot sit still for a second. I have never sat down in my house and felt at home. I suffer with crippling imposter syndrome. Deep down I don't believe I have all that I have. I feel that one day someone is going to tell me to fuck off. I have a pathological fear of failure. To me making a mistake is an act of failure so I never let things lie until I have convinced myself that it is perfect and since perfection doesn't exist, I am haunted. I want the life that everyone else has. I don't want to spend the rest of my life working like a dog. I want to find people who care about me, but at the back of my mind I think no one can love me just being me. I don't even know who I am or what I would be doing if I wasn't the golden child.

People look at me and my lifestyle and think I am living the dream. Yes, that is true if you are into all the trappings that come with a six figure salary. I may come across as confident and on top of my game but inside I am an empty shell. I have no clue who I am and why I am doing all this shit. I am a machine. I keep going achieving and accumulating but at my core I am alone and lost. It's the weirdest thing. I am here physically but I am not here".

Fosia was handed the talking stick.

"I come from a small village in North Africa. My family sent me to London to study, get a good job and send money back home. When I saw him in my study class and realised that he was from

back home, I can't tell you how happy I was. There was a person who knew my language, my food and my traditions. We became inseparable. I introduced him to my family and they hated him on sight. I couldn't understand it at the time. Maybe they could smell his psychopathy way back then. After college our relationship fizzled out. I got married and he disappeared. A couple of years ago, I can't remember exactly, I was doing a bit of shopping and lo and behold I bumped into him. I couldn't believe my eyes. It was so good to see him. That's when the relationship took off. We became lovers. To me it wasn't cheating or at least that's what I told myself. To me it was just like old times. It felt wrong and right at the same time. I would go to the mosque on Friday, church on Sunday to confess my sins and be in a hotel room with him by Monday lunchtime. I didn't stop to think about what I was doing. I was giddy for him. I don't know what happened to me. Maybe I just wanted to feel like a woman and not someone's mum or a wife. I just wanted someone to see me and listen to me.

We met every Monday for a drink and sex. That was the pattern and that was our routine. One day he told me that he was in trouble. He needed money. He had never asked me for money before. I gave him forty thousand pounds of my husband's hard earned cash, my children's college funds and our retirement money. I can't get over the fact that I was so dumb. I gave him the money, we had a few Mondays together and then some Mondays he wouldn't show up. On those Mondays when he didn't show up, I would go into a deep depression. He started to ask for more and more money. I would give it to him just to stay in his good books. I was actually paying him to be with me. I didn't know anything about narcissism or psychopaths. I just didn't want to believe that this guy that I knew virtually all my life had scammed me. Eventually the money ran out. I told him that I had no money left and he told me that if I didn't give him more money he would tell my husband. He sent me a photo of me in the nude. When I received that photo, I thought I was going to have a heart attack. All my thoughts and emotions turned to mush. I couldn't sleep, eat or think straight.

I have been a complete fool. I am so ashamed of myself. I have no words. I gave all my children's inheritance money to a fool. I may as well have flushed it down the toilet. Do you know the amount of times my children have asked for things over the years and I told them 'no'. Why? I wanted them to know the value of money. Yet when this imbecile asked for money, I gave it to him. Look what I did. Look what I did. I am not sure if I can recover from this. I am a fifty three year old woman with five children and I willingly and stupidly gave all our money away to an arse wipe. I never swear and now this fool has me swearing. I thought that I was connecting with the man I had met over thirty years ago. I wanted to go back to those carefree times when we were laughing together in college. I couldn't believe the man he has become. I feel ridiculous. I feel ashamed. I let myself and my children down".

"Let's talk about shame. All of you that have had any dealings with a narcissist will feel shame. It goes with the territory. You feel embarrassed for getting involved in the first place and then for not being able to walk away. Even if it's your parents who are the narcissists, you feel ashamed. If it's your ex-partner, you feel ashamed. You don't know what you did wrong but you must have done something to unleash abuse such as what you have had to endure. According to the psychologist David Hawkins, shame is the lowest of all the emotions you can experience. Feeling ashamed of yourself is close to dying. In fact there is a saying 'I nearly died of shame' as feeling ashamed is like dying. You feel numb. It is a dense, stagnant emotion that renders you hopeless and helpless.

Other emotions come and go. One day you feel sad the next day not so bad. Shame is stagnant energy. It lurks in the recesses of your mind stunting your ability to move on. All relationships with a narcissist are shaming, humiliating and degrading in the end. If you don't think so then you are not at the end.

Tell me Fosia, if one of your best friends told you the story you just told us what would you do?"

"I would listen and support them as much as I could".

"I think it's a shame that you cannot offer the same compassion that you would give to a friend."

"How would you act if your shame didn't exist?"

"I wouldn't care what he said about me. I know who I am. I wouldn't care about what other people thought of me because those who are my real friends know who I am. I wouldn't be upset about the money because I am the one who made that money and I am the one who can make that money again. I wouldn't be worried about my children either because I have given them love and attention from the moment they were born. I told them over and over again that money can't buy love and happiness. I guess I will have to put my money where my mouth especially now that I don't have any in the bank".

She smiled at her play on words. They smiled.

"What keeps you trapped in the abuse is shame. You take full responsibility for how you were treated and accept it as if it was your fault. How fucked up is that? Furthermore you give the shame power because you have kept what happened to you a secret. Why? Because you are ashamed.

But I am here to tell you that abuse of any form or fashion was never your fault. If you accept shame then you are saying that the narcissist was justified in abusing you. If you accept responsibility on behalf of the narcissist then you have sentenced yourself to be a victim for the rest of your life, no matter what you do.

I want you to reject that shit because it just isn't true. I want you all to know that you have nothing to be ashamed of. Hopefully by telling your story and hearing the stories of others you can see that the story of narcissistic abuse is the same. Same shit different day. The narcissist hates exposure. By keeping their abuse a secret and accepting the blame we are actually colluding with them. Tell your story and shame the devil. Bring your story to the light and you will find that it has no power.

Shame is a useless emotion and a waste of time. It is painful to tell your story. I get it. You think that people will judge you. Some people will. Those people are not your tribe. Move on until you find people who are the same as you. Empathetic. Kind. Supportive. Find people who are human and who have a pulse.

The act of telling your story releases the stagnant energy of shame. Story telling is like abuse letting. It is like a valve. In telling your side of the story you detach from the trauma. You are not the trauma, you are not traumatic and you refuse to let any trauma define you.

You have told your story here today and we have listened. With the greatest of respect to all of you, your stories suck. How long do you want the story of abuse to be running on repeat in your head? It's time to tell a different story. A story of survival.

You should feel like a great weight has been lifted from your shoulders. It has. Congratulations everyone for showing up and being your authentic selves. I am sure you are all exhausted.

Let's head back to the resort now before it starts to rain. No sooner had Bev said the word 'rain' and it started to rain. They all let out a squeal and sprang into action. Putting the rubbish in a bag, folding the sun loungers and gathering up their belongings.

"Don't forget to get your treatments tonight. It is your last night, so enjoy it". No one was listening to her.

They ran along the beach. VJ ran into the sea, splashing and laughing like a child and they all followed. Shrieking, laughing and crying tears of freedom.

VJ started to chant.

"I was chained but now I'm free

You're a narc and that don't bother me

I was chained and now I'm free

I was chained and now I'm free

You're a narc and that don't bother me

You're a narc and that don't bother me"

THURSDAY

- GROUP CHAT
- SELF ESTEEM
- NO CONTACT
- THE FINAL WORDS

"Good morning.

I trust you are well.

Yesterday was such a cool day. You dealt with some heavy shit. So let's have some feedback. What did you learn? How do you feel? What are you going to do next?"

After a long pause...

"Yesterday was one of the most amazing experiences of my life. I felt alive for the first time ever. I learnt that it wasn't me. It was never me. I wasn't the crazy one. I was the only sane one in my family. So I was singled out. I get it now. Not because there was anything wrong me, no because there was everything wrong with them. Do you know what's funny? I spent the best part of my life trying to appease the fuckers. I wanted to be one of them. I used to make jokes at my own expense even though I was dying inside just to make them laugh. But now I am glad that I failed

at fitting in and being accepted by them. I am glad that I am the one who is sensitive. I am glad that I am the one who is kind and considerate. I am the one who actually thinks about others and I am glad. My next step is to find a way to distance myself from the madness".

"I feel great. Listening to other people's stories yesterday was so heartening. I didn't feel embarrassed or ashamed to tell my story or to listen to your stories. I felt honoured that you would trust me to witness such delicate information. I know how it felt to tell your story because I told mine. My story is your story and your story is my story. It's same shit different narcissist".

"I don't know where I am. I feel good, don't get me wrong. Yet at the back of my mind I know that I have to go home and deal with the narcissist. I am scared that everything that I have learnt this week is going to fly out the window when I am confronted with them. I really don't know what to think right now. I don't know how I am going to get away from them. I think my next move is to come up with a plan, save some money and buy a big suitcase".

"That sounds like a great plan".

"I feel good. I needed the bodywork, that's for sure. I was so surprised how much stress I had locked up in my body. I recognise that if you have children with a narcissist you are never physically free. That's as it should be. I will

always be there to do the school run, go to sports days or any event for that matter. I will take care of her financially and she will want for nothing. What I will not be doing is allowing her to get in my head. I need to detach from the drama, mentally and spiritually. I can see now that she wants to create a scene. She wants me to feel frustrated because that's how she gets her kicks and she still feels as if she has control over me. She did but not anymore. She cannot control my mind unless I give her permission. I also had a lightbulb moment when I realised that my son is actually 50% my son. I know it sounds crazy but I had given all the power and control to her. I was obsessed with her every move. So much so that I took my eye off my son. My ex can take me for every penny I have but she can never take away the fact that my son is my son. I realise that I in fact have more influence over his development because I am the consistent one. I am the one that he can rely on come hell or come high water. I am the one that can instil in him strong values that can counter the superficial nonsense his mother wants to expose him to. I am his father and I am not going to be a 'weaselly' father. I want to be able to look my son in the eye and be proud that I did the right thing and I did things right. I used to dread picking him up from his mother's but now I can't wait to get back. Bring it on...bring it on".

They sat around chatting for an hour or so. Bev liked them chatting. It gave her an opportunity to assess the group and see what gaps they may still have in their knowledge and understanding. She knew she had to instil in them that the course was not the end or the solution. The course was just the beginning. Very soon they would go back into their worlds and put what they had learnt into practice and it would be a case of trial and error. Did they have the right mindset to meet the challenges and obstacles that they would undoubtably face?

"Before coming here I felt nothing but shame, humiliation and guilt. I told you all my story and none of you judged me. None of you offered me some half-baked advice. All you did was listen without prejudice. So I didn't have to second guess what you might think of me. I didn't have to counter your comments or come up with excuses. As I was talking I heard a little voice say 'You are the one that made the money you lost'. It didn't make sense at the time. One thing I have learnt here is to stay with your emotions. You feel what you feel for a reason. Why is it that when we feel hungry or thirsty we do something about it yet when we feel bad we ignore it? How far would we get if we ignored hunger. So the next time the sentence came into my head I stuck with it. The answer came to me and it was so simple it made me smile. I was the one who made all the money I gave to the narcissist. I made it. It doesn't belong to my children. It was my money. I told myself that it was all about the money but it wasn't the money. It was my shame. The shame of allowing

myself to be taken in like this. I told my story and it is such a relief to get my side of the story off my chest. He tried to turn my community against me. I couldn't go out because I was afraid of what people might say. Honestly some days I thought that people were looking right through me. They could read my mind and see my self-loathing. Now I am going to hold my head up high. I don't give a damn what people think. My duty as a parent is not to save up money that they can have when I die. My duty as a parent is to be a mother. I have always nurtured and supported my children in everything they do. I will continue to do so. That is my legacy. As far as the money is concerned, I was the one who made the money in the first place and if I so wish I can make the money back again. I know if I was to sit down and tell my children my story they would call me all kinds of names and then they would forgive me. I know this to be the case because I raised them to be decent human beings. I guess now what I need to do is learn to forgive myself. I think it will take some time but I am ready".

"I must admit that I came on this workshop to gather as much information as possible so that I could somehow manage the relationship. Yet every time you spoke about the cycle of abuse I couldn't lie to myself anymore. I was well and truly in the cycle. When I listened to all your stories yesterday, I realised that you were telling me my future. That there is no way you can control a narcissist. I admit that I love him. But the love

I have for him is an obsession, it isn't healthy. I think I need help to deal with my addiction. My next step is to find a good therapist who knows about these things and who can support me".

"Thank you for sharing. I know it can't have been easy to bare your souls like that. It takes courage. You did it. Congratulations. There are many reasons why you feel the way that you do now. For some of you it is the first time that you have been listened to and taken seriously. That is validation in itself. For others you spoke your truth and unburdened yourselves of guilt and shame. I myself feel privileged to hear your stories. The trust that you have in me and each other to bear witness to your pain and to believe that we would not further abuse you is humbling. I want you to hold on to the moment of storytelling because actually it is truth telling. The truth shall set you free.

So now what? What are you going to do with the rest of your life?

Now that you have got rid of all that toxic energy that was running around in your system and spoiling your fun, you are free to be whoever you want to be.

Who will you be?

So what do we know? The narcissist is not capable of love. You are. You have the capacity for deep and true love. They don't. So don't go looking for love in all the wrong places and don't give your love away to people who wouldn't know what love was if it bit them on the shoulder.

You have the ability to feel true and beautiful emotions, like happiness. The narcissist cannot feel happiness unless they are fucking up someone else's happiness. It is you who has the capacity to connect with others, to sprinkle kindness and joy. The narcissist can only dream about such things or view it on Netflix.

You are the opposite of the narcissist. You are light and they are dark. They tried to steal your light. Tell me now, are you going to allow them to succeed? I hope you realise that you are the one with the power. When you shine light into a dark room, the light will brighten up the darkest of rooms. You cannot do the opposite.

The only way to get over narcissistic abuse from childhood or in adulthood is to work on yourself. A narcissist cannot change, they are trapped in the cesspit of who they are. You, on the other hand, can change. You have the power of self-reflection. It is oh too easy to see yourself as the victim. Don't do that. If you fall into a victim reality you will see the world as a dangerous place, where people are not to be trusted and are only out to get you. If you become a victim then you may as well put a crown on the narcissist's head. They win and you lose. If you let the narcissist win that means they control your every thought and your every move forever. When you identify as a victim the world will treat you accordingly. You will wind up in situations and with people who confirm what you think of yourself back to you. It is the Law of Cause and Effect.

It is important to develop boundaries. Strong boundaries are what you need to protect your self-esteem and your mental wellbeing. Think about boundaries like this: you have skin to protect your physical body so nothing gets in and your internal organs don't spill out and bleed all over the place. You need mental and emotional boundaries to protect who you are from outside forces which may not have your best interests at heart.

Ask yourself 'who am I?' Ask yourself 'Who am I not?' See what comes up for you. You will never be able to be an individual in your own right if you don't know who you are.

Many people have defined you and made assumptions based on their definitions. Maybe it's time for you to define or redefine yourself. If you do not define yourself then don't complain if people define you for you. If you do not know who you are then there is nothing to protect. If there is nothing to protect then there can be no boundaries. How can I put it: in order for there to be a boundary around a field there has to be a field for the boundary to go around.

If you say that you are a person of integrity, for example, then you have to be it and live it. Your boundaries should be clear to you first of all and to all those around you. You should be able to detect when people are not acting with integrity and you have to develop the courage to move on, quickly. Every time you give people second chances or turn a blind eye you are weakening your own boundaries. You have to learn to put yourself first. It isn't selfish, it is essential. You are no good to anyone, not even yourself if you are a traumatised victim.

The cornerstone of healthy strong boundaries is self-esteem. Self-esteem is what you think of yourself deep down. It stands to reason that if you think highly of yourself then your self-esteem will be high. High self-esteem means you respect yourself and you don't allow people to take liberties with you. When you have high self-esteem no one can tell you anything about yourself that you don't already know. You don't need anyone to tell you how amazing you are. You already know. You don't need anyone to complete you. You are already complete and you are the real deal.

You want someone to complement you. To enjoy you with you. If someone isn't adding joy to your sweet self and your rich experiences of life on this planet then they can just get lost. You are not broken you and you do not need fixing. You sure as hell do not need someone without a soul defining you and then getting off on hurting you.

Albert Einstein famously said:

"God does not play dice with the universe".

You are not an accident or a mistake. You are as you should be. You are perfect. When I talk about working on yourself people have a hard time understanding what this means. It means treating yourself like buried treasure that has been excavated and restored to its original glory.

There is nothing missing. You are complete. You are the full package. If the person in front of you cannot see that, then that's too bad. Self- esteem means accepting yourself the way you are. Yes, you could be taller, thinner, smarter, and richer and maybe you're not any of those things but you love yourself anyway.

No one can give you self-esteem. That is your job. Maybe you thought for a second that the narcissist could give you the self-esteem you never had. The narcissist cannot give you what they do not have. The narcissist cannot hack it because they are empty inside. That's why they need you. When your self-esteem is high then it is not in your interests to put others down or make their lives a misery. By their actions you can see that the narcissist is full of self-loathing and all they want to do is share the pain.

A high self-esteem is like repellent to a narcissist. They cannot and will not stick around if they know you know who you are and you like who you are. They will not be able to get to you so to speak if they discover that you have strong healthy boundaries. They cannot survive if you know your worth and what you are is priceless. Self-esteem is like having a black belt in emotional intelligence.

When you have a black belt no one is going to pick a fight with you unless they are a complete idiot.

Ask yourself this question:

"What in the world would I be doing if I had not encountered the narcissist?"

Make a list. That list is now your new bucket list.

- Do something that takes you outside of your comfort zone. Whenever you catch yourself saying 'Oh I could never do that' that is the exact thing you should be doing. It doesn't matter what you do as long as you do something.

- Take dance classes. You may not be invited to Dancing with the Stars but you will be able to shake your groove thing at your next birthday party. Join a swimming class or a cycle class. Again you may not be called up for the next Olympics but you will feel the benefits to your health.

- Learn a skill. Take up a hobby. Take a class. See the world one country at a time.

It is important for you to keep moving physically, mentally and spiritually. Your movements become your rituals and your rituals become your new habits and your new habits become your way of life.

Break

You may remember the story I told you on Tuesday about Narcissus, the boy in Greek mythology who fell in love with his reflection and died. I feel I can now tell you the rest of the story.

Nemesis is the goddess of revenge and it was she who lured Narcissus to the river and to his death. The goddess Nemesis knew that Narcissus was self-absorbed and that was his Achilles heel, so she knew how to destroy him.

The Achilles heel of the narcissist you are dealing with is rejection. The narcissist needs to realise that you do not care what they to do, what they say about you or who they send to terrorise you. When you cut off all means of supply they wither and die.

'No contact' is the term we use for this in narcissist circles. I want to tell you what it isn't before I tell you what it is.

Some people think that going 'no contact' is something they do for a week or two to teach the narcissist a lesson. I saw a video on YouTube that declared that if you go 'no contact' for twenty days then the narcissist will come back to you. Then I saw another video claiming that if you go 'no contact' for forty days, no, sixty days the narcissist will beg to come back. This is manipulative bullshit. If you want to play those games then you are in good company. The narcissist is a master manipulator. Good luck!

Some people go 'no contact' thinking that they are giving the narcissist a taste of their own medicine. You cannot teach a narcissist a lesson.

All teachable moments will go straight over their heads because they do not have the capacity for self-reflection.

Some people think that 'no contact' is a matter of blocking the narcissist on social media and changing your mobile number. It is more than that. 'No contact' means that the narcissist no longer has access to you. You are dead to them and they are dead to you.

Some people struggle with 'no contact' because of the trauma bond. It is tough and probably the hardest thing you'll ever have to do. Going 'no contact' is like going cold turkey. I want you to know that every time you go 'no contact' and give in you are showing the narcissist exactly how much shit you can take and still go back to them. I can tell you this: every time you go back the abuse will be worse.

Going 'no contact' it is a choice. It means that you choose you over the narcissist. You may not realise it at the time but the narcissist realises it straight away. They are dying and that is why they send all kinds of flying monkey tactics your way.

In order to go 'no contact' you must disappear from the face of the earth as far as the narcissist is concerned and you must remove every trace of the narcissist from your life. When I say everything, I mean everything.

You block them from your phone, social media and from all aspects of your life. You take their name off anything that you shared together. Bills, contracts and memberships. You pack up all their belongings and send them back to them, give it to charity or throw it away. If you do not know what to do with their stuff send it to their mother. My point is get rid of it. All the things they bought for you or for the house, get rid of it. There must be no reminders of them in your energy field.

Going 'no contact' is an action. It is the art of fighting without fighting. You remove yourself mind, body and soul from the relationship. To me 'no contact' is an act of defiance. People think that 'no contact' doesn't work because they are not there to see the narcissist suffer. You do not need to see them suffer. Believe me when I tell you 'no contact' is like death to the narcissist. When they have no access to you, they cannot play with your emotions which means no supply. This to the narcissist is abandonment all over again. It is the feeling of being abandoned and rejection that made a narcissist a narcissist in the first place. When you pull the plug on them they will go into a frenzy. They will try every trick in their book to get you back again. When you go 'no contact' do not be surprised to be hoovered up, love bombed and bombarded. Do not be concerned and do not give in. It is just the antics of a desperate creepy crawly being flushed down the toilet trying to latch on to something to save its own life.

'No contact' is a process. When you cut off all ties with the narcissist you are going to be left with a tsunami of emotions. All the emotions that you have denied for so long will come rushing in. You may feel anger, sadness, depression and stupidity and not necessarily in that order. You might feel that you are going crazy without them. You are not. What you are going through is withdrawal symptoms. Keep going!

The brilliant psychologist Elizabeth Kobler Ross developed what is known as the grief model. She stated that anyone who experiences loss in any form or fashion will experience grief. Kobler Ross was looking at the loss of someone who has died but calling time on a narcissist is a form of death to you. You will go through shock, denial, anger, depression and sadness. All your emotions will surface when the coast is clear for them to be dealt with. Do not be afraid since this is an opportunity to heal. I know that it is terrifying to face your emotions. But know this also: your emotions didn't kill you then and they will not kill you now. What doesn't kill you is bound to make you stronger. All your emotions want is to be listened to, validated and respected. Pretending that shit didn't happen when it obviously did happen is not treating yourself with respect. Giving other people the benefit of the doubt isn't treating yourself with respect. Listening to bullshit that insults your intelligence is not respecting yourself. Allowing the narcissist to criticise you, judge you, define you, walk all over you and at the same time feed off you is not treating yourself with respect. Denying your feelings is not treating yourself with respect. If you are angry then be angry.

You have a right to be angry. Let your anger be heard until it is no more. Only when you let go of all the negative stuff can there be any space for the positive stuff. According to Kobler Ross, only when you fearlessly deal with each emotion will you reach a place of acceptance. You will come to see that none of the shit that happened to you had anything to do with you. You just happened to be there at the time.

'No contact' depends on your circumstances. Some people can walk and not look back and some people cannot.

Do not beat yourself up if you cannot go 'the full monty' with 'no contact'. Do what you can and what you think is right for you rather than what you think other people want you to do. 'No contact' can be a physical thing but in many circumstances a physical 'no contact' is desirable but not possible. If you cannot go 'no contact' physically then you need to do the next best thing. You need to go 'no contact' mentally.

You might love to go 'no contact' with an elderly parent, but you can't as you are responsible for them. 'No contact' in this situation might mean that you outsource as much as you can to agencies who are well practised in such situations. Set up systems with the necessary agencies such as carers and home visits of all description. When you visit protect your boundaries by not getting into any debates, discussions or arguments about anything. If your parent insists on pushing your boundaries then you get up say 'farewell' and leave.

If you have children with a narcissist then clearly 'no contact' isn't an option. If you thought that co-parenting with a narcissist was going to work then I guess you didn't think it through. Co-parenting suggests cooperating. The narcissist will never cooperate with you even at the expense of their own children. Every day is a battlefield. It will be even worse if they know that you are anxious about your children being with them. They will go out of their way to upset you. If you want your child to eat healthily then the narcissist will feed them junk food, just to get at you. Whatever you request the narcissist to do they will do the opposite. They know that if they can upset you then they still control you.

Co-parenting with a narcissist is frustrating beyond belief so try parallel parenting instead. Parallel parenting means that you parent alongside each other and the interactions between you are limited and formal. When you decide to go down the parallel parenting route then everything is conducted via email. In that way everything is recorded and you have evidence should the matter need to go to court in the future. Recording everything in and of itself should make the narcissist watch their step a little. Narcissists hate rules and regulations.

Where possible make sure that someone else is there to hand over or receive the child. It could be a friend or a neighbour. Make yourself scarce. In that way they cannot say anything to you to wind you up.

Lastly don't be concerned if they give your child junk food, just make up for it when they get home. Do not be concerned if the narcissist tries to buy the child's love and affection. Do not compete. Instead when the child is in your care take them to an animal sanctuary or get them doing some voluntary work. If the narcissist wants to influence your child in order to get back at you, do not take the bait. Do not make a fuss or fight. Your protestations are giving them too much information on how to get to you. When you have a child with a narcissist it is not so much a case of 'no contact', it is more a case of 'no comment'. If you have to make contact keep your communication to a bare minimum. I don't mean being rude. It's just if they ask you a question answer the question and move on. Do not engage. If you are living with the narcissist then separate everything out as much as possible. Do your own washing. Buy your own milk. In that way you will not be drawn into petty arguments. The mindset you need to adopt is one of living with a stranger. This sounds easy for me to say but it is tough. There is no magic solution to this. If you are entangled with a narcissist then learn mental resilience. In the words of the late great Bruce Lee, you need to 'be like water'. You have to learn emotional martial arts and mental gymnastics.

'No contact' is the best option when dealing with a narcissist. But if you can't go full 'no contact' then use the next few techniques to develop mental toughness. They are grey rocking, fogging and broken record. I know the names sound crazy but they are very effective.

Grey rocking is the art of fighting back without fighting. Instead of giving the narcissist supply you turn into a rock. You can't get blood out of a stone and you can't get supply out of a grey rock.

This is how you do it:

Give them nothing to go on. If they ask you a question instead of answering directly say "eh" "umm". This will annoy the narcissist. That is the whole idea. If the supply dries up the narcissist will have to go elsewhere and leave you alone.

Disengage and disconnect. Do not give them any eye contact. If they try to drag you into an argument, leave the room or change the subject.

If you have to speak to them then keep your answers short. Say 'yes', 'no' or 'let me get back to you'. Stop giving explanations.

Do not tell them anything. If they ask you what you are up to, tell them politely you have no plans. If you tell a narcissist anything about what you are doing then you can bet your bottom dollar that they will set about sabotaging them.

Fogging: also known as agreeing and amplifying any true elements in what the narcissist says but not in the way that they expect. The big idea is that you give the narcissist nothing to latch on to. It is very difficult to argue with someone who agrees with you all the time.

Here a few examples of how it works:

Agree with the narcissist. If they say:

"You're wearing that shirt again today". You could say in response.

"That's right. I'm wearing that shirt again."

Agree with the possibility or probability of any criticism they hurl at you. Do not get defensive.

If they say: *"You're so messy"* you might reply,

"You could be right about that."

Agree with any logic in what they say. Do not be drawn in to their fuzzy logic.

If they say: *"I need a new mobile. If you buy me one then I won't have to use this piece of crap"*.

You say "You're right. A new mobile would be nice".

Agree with any opportunity for you to improve and grow. Do not take anything personally. They say: *"You drive like a maniac"*. Your response could be something like this, "Yes...I should watch my speed at times".

Broken record is a technique that enables you to ask for what you want and stick to your guns without being drawn into any manipulative traps.

This is how it works.

You: "I want you to pick the children up at 5 pm tonight as they need to do their homework and be in bed by 9pm".

Them: *"I can't possibly be there to pick them up at 5, the traffic is awful at that hour".*

You: "I do agree that the traffic can be awful but I need you to pick the children up at 5 pm".

Them: *"Well you can talk you never pick the children up on time when I've got them".*

You: "Yes I agree I have been late on the rare occasion but I would like you to pick the children up at 5 pm to night so they can do their homework and be in bed by 9 pm".

Them: *"Can't you ask your mother to pick them up if it is so important to you?"*

You: "I will ask my mother on another occasion. On this occasion I want you to pick the children up at 5pm".

When you are using the broken record technique. You do not sway, deviate or get dragged down a rabbit hole. You simply ask for what you want and stick to it. It is important to listen to what the narcissist is saying so you can reflect that in your response. "I know the traffic is heavy but this is what I want". "I appreciate that I could ask my mother but I am asking you". If you use the broken record technique the narcissist will quickly run out of retorts. They don't have a lot of imagination so it shouldn't take long for them to realise that you are not there to play their game.

Negative enquiry is a technique you can use to deflect criticisms and abuse. This is a powerful technique because instead of soaking up the criticism as you usually would, you face it head on, acknowledge it and challenge the narcissist. Challenging their opinions and criticism of you is going to shock the narcissist and leave them flabbergasted. Emotional intelligence is not their thing.

Let me give you an example of how it works:

Let's say the narcissist criticises your clothes.

Them: *"Your clothes are awful. You look an absolute mess. I am not going out with you looking like that"*.

You: "You say my clothes are awful and I look a mess. Can you tell me what exactly it is that you do not like about my clothes?"

I guarantee you they will not have an answer.

Practise these techniques and become good at them. I have given you four techniques so you can mix them up. I suggest that you start off small. Use them in areas of your life where the consequences are minimal before you proceed to using them on the narcissist.

These are emotional intelligence techniques so they work in any situation. The really powerful thing about these techniques is that you can't get them wrong. Just attempting to do them disrupts the narcissistic cycle of abuse. The more you disrupt the cycle the weaker the cycle becomes. The narcissist becomes discombobulated. They are not getting their supply in the usual way. If they can't get supply they will not stick around. Let me rephrase that: if the narcissist cannot get supply from you they cannot stick around. Just like a vampire needs blood to stay alive the narcissist needs supply to survive.

We are now at the end of our time together. You now know a lot about the narcissist. But don't make it your life's work to understand the narcissist. You know enough to get by.

Now that we are at the end of the workshop, I want to leave you with this thought. It may not sit right with some of you now but hopefully if you keep working on yourself, my words will make sense one day.

Maybe the narcissist came into your life for a reason. What was that reason? Maybe the narcissist came into your life to create a situation where you can be healed. Maybe they opened up wounds of childhood abuse that needed to be dealt with. Deal with them now. Don't let your feelings go underground again. Get yourself a good therapist. Even if you didn't suffer child abuse maybe the narcissist entered your life to show you that the way you were living your life wasn't working. Maybe you needed to learn the hard way to fall in love with yourself first and foremost.

My hope for you is that one day you will be so at peace with what happened that you actually thank the narcissist and get on with it. I hope that you recognise that you are complete in and of yourself. You are the real deal. You have what the narcissist can only dream of. You are fully human. I hope you open your heart to the possibilities of finding love if that is what you want. There are still some really good people out there waiting to meet you. You will know that you're healed when you realise that the narcissist came into your life for a reason ant the reason was to help you heal. When you make this realisation the narcissist will have no power over you. The cycle of abuse is broken and you will be free to walk your own path.

I wish you all a safe journey home....

2 YEARS LATER

Bev walked along the beach towards the cove. She must give the cove a name one day. It deserves a name she thought. It had witnessed a lot of suffering. Thank God it had witnessed a lot of healing too. No one comes away from the cove without some sort of transformation.

She arrived at the cove ready with sage and crystals. Bev liked to clear the space the day before the workshop began because she knew she wouldn't get a chance once the workshop started.

She was surprised to see the resort staff there.

"Hi there...Que pasa...what's up....?"

"Hola senorita, we are setting up the cove for an event this afternoon".

"Can't you set up a few metres away from here? This is the place that I like to prepare for my workshop. I don't want to run a workshop with empty beer bottles and half eaten chicken wings."

"Lo siento...we have been instructed to set the party up right here in the cove".

Bev sighed. What could she do?

The sage and the crystals were going to be useless after everyone had trampled through them.

"Ahhh. I am going to have to come back early tomorrow morning to purify this space". She thought.

"What time does this party start?"

"It starts in about 20 minutes. All we are doing is adding the final touches. Musica, drinks, flowers. That's it!"

The staff busied themselves with their duties. They lit candles and lanterns. They lay gemstones of citrine, sapphire and tourmaline in the sand. They cast flowers around the makeshift tables and chairs.

Bev couldn't believe her eyes. Everything was all yellow.

It was beautiful. She let out a gasp. She was brought back to the present moment by the spluttering sounds of a walkie talkie. Apparently the party was on its way and due to arrive in ten minutes.

"Well, I better make myself scarce", she muttered to herself. I do not want to gatecrash the party.

It suddenly dawned on her that the only way back to the resort was the way she had come and that meant that she would have to walk through the crowd.

She couldn't think of anything worse. She had her worst outfit on. She made a promise to herself that if she ever got back to the resort the first thing she would do was throw away the clothes she was wearing. She realised that she had ducked out of the resort without even combing her hair properly. This was going to be painful. She didn't want to do the walk of shame back to the resort.

She knew the staff well. "Can I hitch a lift back to the resort with one of you? I am not really dressed for a party."

As soon as the words left her lips she realised that it was too late. The crowd was nearly upon her. Oh no!

Maybe no one would notice her and she could skulk around in the background and then disappear.

She could make out like she was a guest but it would be hard to pull it off wearing joggers and the tee-shirt she had slept in.

She watched the party arrive. They were singing, dancing and cheering. A couple seemed to be the centre of attention and they wore garlands of yellow around their necks. Someone sure loves yellow.

Oh so it's a wedding party. Great!

She watched them as they drew nearer. They were having a good time. What caught Bev's attention was the laughter. They were so joyous. It was mesmerising. As thy came closer Bev had an out of body experience. She was familiar with out of body experiences through meditation but she wasn't used to having one when her eyes were wide open. She blinked. A member of staff handed her a drink. She drunk it. It was tequila. What the hell's going on?

She had stepped into a parallel universe. It took a moment for her brain to adjust. Wait a minute! She knew them. She knew them but she couldn't place them. Her brain was doing cartwheels.

How did she know them? Why did they decide to hold their wedding at her cove?

Everyone was a sight to behold all decked out in various shades of yellow. The yellow of their outfits against the yellow of the sun and the sand was breathtaking. This was going to be a good celebration she thought.

She was surrounded by people, all smiling at her.

She was in shock. For once Bev had nothing to say.

Heading up the party was VJ and Harshida. They were *still* holding hands. Bev was unable to close her mouth. They laughed.

"We are getting married today. Here at the cove. You, dear Bev are the guest of honour."

The words bounced off her brain, more cartwheels.

Someone brought her another drink and someone else gave her a yellow kaftan to wear. They sat down.

"After we left the workshop VJ and I stayed in touch. I called him whenever I was struggling with my husband who is now my ex".

VJ took up the story:

"... and I texted Harshida if I was having trouble with my family.

It was our escape. We started fantasising about running away. Not together at first. The fantasy was what kept us alive. When one of us was down the other one would raise the other's spirits, by talking about our fantasy. The fantasy was a blank canvas and every time we talked we filled it in a little bit more. The fantasy became really real. We talked and talked about making the fantasy real. We didn't realise that our fantasy was really an exit strategy.

One day Harshida texted to tell me that Raj had beaten her up yet again. This time I saw red. I couldn't stand the thought of her taking another beating from that monster. I was bursting with rage.

I went to her house. I drove for hours to get there. He opened the door. It was all I could to do to stop myself sucker punching him. I looked past him and saw Harshida cowering in the corner. She was shaking. I don't know what got into me, I pushed past this mountain of a man and went to Harshida. He could have killed me but I didn't care. I scooped her up in my arms and carried her out the front door. Raj stood there not knowing what to do so he started shouting. All the neighbours were out, craning their necks to see what all the commotion was about.

Raj rushed to block our path..."

"Hey what do you think you're doing...put my wife down".

He was practically screaming and shouting to people to help him. I was intent on getting Harshida in the car.

"He's abducting my wife...help me...somebody call the police".

I turned and spoke to him but loud enough for everyone to hear.

"Listen I know what you are. You are a narcissist. In fact the 'n' word is too mild for people like you. You are a predator that feeds off the misery you cause. Does it make you feel big, eh? Do you feel like a real man when you beat up a defenceless woman? What gives you the right to think that you can terrorise someone to the point where they give up the will to live? You are despicable. You are a slug. People think you live here in this nice house on this nice street with nice neighbours but really you live under a stone. You are a taker, a user and an abuser. You are the armpit of humanity. A malfunction. A flipping

abomination. It stops here and now. DO YOU HEAR ME?

You have been abusing this woman for too long. I am taking Harshida to the hospital. If any of you help him or try to stop me then know that you are aiding and abetting a monster.

I am going to get her checked out by a doctor. For your sake, she better be OK, if not I am coming back and I will rip you a new arsehole.

Listen to me, the next time you hear from her it will be to sign divorce papers. You will sign these papers without hesitation. If you don't she will come for you and I will be right behind her. I will use the medical reports from previous hospital visits to make sure that you end up in jail. Your new arse will come in very handy there. Karma is a bitch and she doesn't like to see one of her own being beaten up by a fuck pig like you.

The man who you think is a respected member of the community is a wife beater. He loves porn and tries out the techniques on his wife. When she refuses he beats her".

"He's lying...he's lying. I have never seen this man before in my life".

"It was all Raj could say. He was actually pleading with the neighbours not to listen to me. We were at an impasse. It looked like he wasn't going to let us go.

At that moment Harshida lifted her jumper. She didn't care who saw her. Her entire upper body was covered in bruises. Tell the truth and shame the devil.

Everyone gasped. They were paralysed in shock. I put Harshida in the back seat, made sure her seat belt was fastened and drove away as fast as was legally possible. Neither of us looked back. Neither of us knew where we were going".

VJ paused.

At that moment a hundred yellow balloons were released into the late afternoon sky.

"What's with all the yellow?"

"Ahhhh! We remembered the story of Narcissus and how he fell in love with his own reflection. The narcissus is a beautiful yellow flower, very close to a daffodil. We decided to reclaim the colour. By reclaiming the flower we want to declare that although we have been through the valley of the shadow of death, slept with the enemy and dined with the devil, we are still standing.

We wear yellow because it is the colour of the sun. Everyone loves sunny days. We wear yellow because we are the sun. We wear yellow and sing along to Coldplay. To us yellow is a symbol of unity. For all the people who have had their lives destroyed by a narcissist mother, father, sister, brother, partner, boss or friend, we see you and you are not alone. We take back our power from under the nose of the narcissist. We realise that they are incomplete humans masquerading as humans.

We have been learning over the past two years. The yellow is symbolic. The yellow is the colour of the third chakra in the body. The third chakra or solar plexus chakra is located about four fingers above the navel. An experience with a narcissist is like being kicked in the gut. The solar plexus chakra is the centre of who we are. It houses all of our emotions. It's a good place to start to heal. We have learnt that when emotions come up instead of trying to suppress them it is important to sit with them and dissect them. Emotions do not have power over you unless you give them power.

Whenever we were going through our trauma we would remember your teachings. We remembered you saying that pain was part of the process to healing.

The PTSD was a bitch. It was well and truly in every cell of Harshida's body. We found out to our cost that even though we had escaped our abusers we were still having a shit time of it all. Harshida suffered from flashbacks and horrendous nightmares. I am not going to lie but some nights I thought I was going to lose my life. She screamed like a banshee. I came to realise that this was trauma leaving her body. So we went with it. When she trembled with fear I put my arms around her. When she ranted I was on standby to listen or to pass the tissues. She did the same for me. In the beginning neither of us had any energy. It was the craziest thing. We were both exhausted and yet we couldn't sleep. If we did sleep we would have terrible nightmares. We both were hungry and yet we couldn't eat. The food got stuck in our throats. You'll be pleased to know that we continued with the bodywork. Every morning without fail we went for long walks. Sometimes we swam, other times we danced and we even did cold water showers. We never stopped with the massages. Little by little we began to understand our pain. I saw Harshida's pain and it spoke to my pain. She saw my pain and it spoke to hers. Little by little we healed. Little by little we fell in love. Harshida doesn't judge me in any form or fashion. I felt free for the first time in my life. I could do what I wanted and go where I wanted to go. But the truth was I found that I didn't want to do anything unless it was with Harshida.

I know that she is older than me but I am done trying to fit in with society's views. I have done that most of my life and look where it got me. I am a misfit. Hallelujah!

I see Harshida's spirit. I love her not her age. It took a lot of convincing to get her to marry me but finally she said 'yes'.

The next thing was for her to get a divorce. He signed the divorce papers without too much trouble. I only had to remind him of the conversation we had had in the street a couple of years back.

So after the divorce came through the rest was pretty easy. We knew where we wanted to get married and we know who we wanted to be at the wedding. It had to be in Malta. We knew that you are in Malta around four times a year and so all we had to do was choose one of the dates.

We sent emails out to all your past students. Asia helped us with all the admin. You are right she is an amazing events planner".

Bev looked at Asia in astonishment and Asia raised her glass and an eyebrow at the same time. Cheers!

"The last thing you said to us at the workshop really pissed me off. You said it would piss us off and it did! You said that the narcissist came into our life for a reason and that once we find out the reason and come to terms with the reason then we would have no reason to suffer further. I struggled with that idea. For the love of God I couldn't see any reason for the abuse I'd suffered at the hands of my family.

Harshida and I discussed this many times. No matter what we did we always came back to our trauma and victimhood. So we decided to stop looking for answers, when we didn't even know what the questions were.

In the evenings we would sit and chat about life, our day or whatever. One evening we just started talking about the narcissist coming into our lives for a reason but instead of getting all defensive about it, we decided to explore the possibility. This is what we did.

The first step is to ask yourself 'Who am I?' If you are anything like us we drew a blank. We had no idea who we are. We didn't take it personally. So that was our starting point. We kept on asking the question "who am I" I am telling you that your mind will jump around like a monkey but if you keep asking the question you move beyond your name, profession, gender, sexuality, religion and possessions. You will start to define yourself in terms of your values, attributes, beliefs. You may say things like 'I am an empath?'. These are just words and pretty meaningless at that if you do not walk the talk. So the next step is to ask questions "In what way am I an empath?" In other words how I demonstrate empathy in the world. "What is it about being an empath that I like or how does being an empath feed my soul?" If being an empath is an expression of how I am how can I protect my empathy. We found this an important step. Because being an empath is not about running around saving the world at the expense of yourself. Our empathy, well at least mine, is more targeted. I am no use to anyone if I am battered and bruised. I do the best I can to help others and if it gets too much I know now when to back away".

Harshida took up the story from there.

"I found it difficult to define myself. After years of abuse, I had no clue. So V.J would play this game. Instead of defining what I was, we flipped it and defined the things I was not. So you could say "I am not greedy. So that means you are kind. I am not materialistic". I am a "minimalist". By answering the question who am I or who you are not you are defining or redefining yourself.

Establishing who you are is at the core of healing from abuse. Without knowing who you are you cannot develop self-esteem and without self-esteem you cannot develop boundaries. Defining who you are doesn't have to be perfect. You are a work in progress. Every day you make yourself available to discover who you are.

For me the next step is establishing my values. In other words what is important to me? One value that is important to me is integrity. I do what I say I'm going to do and I like people who do the same. If people do what they say then I know I can trust them. If the evidence shows that the person I am dealing with has no integrity then I stop entertaining them. Integrity is a boundary for me. Integrity is the measure I use to decide who to let in to my life and who to let go. The value of integrity also keeps me in line as well. I have to make sure that my word is my bond otherwise I am lying to myself. It is hypocritical to look for values in others that you are not embodying yourself.

Once you have a working model of who you are then the next step is your beliefs. Your beliefs are simply your point of view. So for example do you believe you are a victim? I did. I had to dismantle that belief. I examined everything that I said or did that colluded or supported that belief. I challenged everything. I didn't allow my mind to get away with a thing. Yes I had been victimised but was I a victim? I decided that I wasn't going to indulge that belief any longer. Being a victim serves no purpose. So I let it go.

As I sifted through the entangled stagnant emotions of my existence and got rid of some shitty beliefs about myself that were no longer true, something magical happened. I had created space to think about what I wanted to do with my life. I was unencumbered and untethered.

I had established my identity, my values and my beliefs. That is the inner work. The outer work is figuring out what you want to do with your life. I did a skills inventory. I wrote down everything that I was good at. If you like doing something chances are you are good at it. Once I had a list, I looked at each skill and broke them down into subskills. In my case I loved to draw. An artist has focus and attention to detail. My ex told me I was talentless every day. I came to a place where I just thought to myself 'who the hell was he to tell me that I had no talent. When did he become an art critic?' I liked drawing and I decided that I was good at it.

Let me tell you, working on yourself is hard work. I went back to art classes after nearly twenty years and loved it. If I was useless at art then I needed a professional to tell me that. It turned out that I was very good. I was so good that I decided to retrain as an art teacher. I worked on my emotional intelligence. The first time I said 'no' to someone without feeling guilty was a joyous day. VJ and I went out to celebrate. We kept growing, learning and having a lot of fun along the way. Reinventing ourselves and distancing ourselves from our past. The more you do the more there is of you to explore".

VJ interjected:

"I joined Harshida for a few drawing classes and they were fun but one day I decided to try out an acting class instead. It was like coming home. I found the answer to my question. Im a good actor. I get a lot of work. Directors tell me that I am easy to work with because I can emote any feeling. I can cry on demand. I didn't need to go to drama school, my family had been my drama school.

I know it is a cliché but we realised that if we hadn't gone through so much trauma with the narcissist we would never have found each other.

You were right. The narcissist doesn't happen to you. The narcissist happens for you. Do you know I actually feel sorry for narcissists now? We are the ones that experience things that the narcissist can only dream about. We are the ones that cry watching soppy movies. We are the ones who are touched by a random act of kindness. We love sunsets. We love connecting with people. We love to sing, and dance and to laugh. What's more, we can laugh at ourselves. We enjoy a good debate. We love children and animals. We are empaths and that is our superpower.

In fact we are everything that the narcissist is not. They can never be us. We are human.

Let's drink to that and let's get married".

And so they did.

When the song came on everyone stopped. They looked around at each other not knowing what to do. They listened. As the words sunk in they started to smile. The smile turned into laughter and the laughter turned into dancing. They sang along at the top of their voices. It was the narcissist slayer's anthem.

(Curtesy of Elton John and Bernie Taulpin)

You could never know what it's like
Your blood like winter freezes just like ice
And there's a cold lonely light that shines from you
You'll wind up like the wreck you hide behind
that mask you use

And did you think this fool could never win?

Well, look at me, I'm coming back again
I got a taste of love in a simple way
And if you need to know while I'm still standing,
you just fade away

Don't you know I'm still standing better than I
ever did
Looking like a true survivor, feeling like a little
kid
I'm still standing after all this time
Picking up the pieces of my life without you on
my mind

I'm still standing (yeah, yeah, yeah)
I'm still standing (yeah, yeah, yeah)

Once I never could have hoped to win
You're starting down the road leaving me again
The threats you made were meant to cut me
down
And if our love was just a circus, you'd be a clown
by now

You know I'm still standing better than I ever did
Looking like a true survivor, feeling like a little
kid
I'm still standing after all this time
Picking up the pieces of my life without you on
my mind

I'm still standing (yeah, yeah, yeah)
I'm still standing (yeah, yeah, yeah)

Don't you know that I'm still standing better
than I ever did?
Looking like a true survivor, feeling like a little
kid
I'm still standing after all this time
Picking up the pieces of my life without you on
my mind

I'm still standing (yeah, yeah, yeah)
I'm still standing (yeah, yeah, yeah)
I'm still standing (yeah, yeah, yeah)
I'm still standing (yeah, yeah, yeah)
I'm still standing (yeah, yeah, yeah)
I'm still standing (yeah, yeah, yeah)

Bev looked around at all the beautiful people.
She was bursting with happiness. Her work here
was done. Tomorrow she had another workshop
to deliver. There was no peace for the narcissist
slayer.